NATURAL HOME
HEALTH CARE
Using
ESSENTIAL OILS

NOTICE

The aim of this book is to inform and thereby serve its readers by introducing them to an understanding of health and hygiene through natural means.

Anyone afflicted by a medical condition should consult their doctor for a diagnosis of the condition and an appropriate choice of measures for its relief.

The authors cannot be held responsible for consequences resulting from not observing the above rule.

© 1998 Daniel Pénoël, MD, and Rose-Marie Pénoël for Osmobiose Publishing.

Éditions Osmobiose 1998
La Drôme, France

Distributed in North America by
Essential Science Publishing
Hurricane, Utah

ISBN No. 2909531-02-3

NATURAL HOME HEALTH CARE *Using* ESSENTIAL OILS

An Introduction to the Theory, Practice, and Technique of Integral Aromatherapy (Osmobiosis)

Daniel Pénoël, MD
and
Rose-Marie Pénoël

Foreword by Abby Bean
Edited by Brian Manwaring

(An American English translation from the
French original titled "Pratique Aromatique Familiale,"
Revised and Enlarged)

COVER DESIGN
AND
PHOTO CREDITS

The artwork displayed on the front and back cover was created by Dr. Pénoël's wife and co-author, Rose-Marie. She designs the cover art used on all books published by Osmobiose Publishing.

All photographs contained in the photo section of this book were arranged for and taken by Dr. Daniel Pénoël and Rose-Marie Pénoël.

OTHER WRITINGS AND CONTRIBUTIONS BY DR. DANIEL PÉNOËL
AND
ROSE-MARIE PÉNOËL

Jean-Paul Tessier et l'Ecole de l'Art Medical
(A la recontre d'une thérapie "vieille comme le monde")
(1976, Higher Doctoral Thesis)

Phytomedicine (in collaboration with Pierre Franchomme) (1980)

L'Aromathérapie exactement (in collaboration with Pierre Franchomme)
(Editions Jollois, 1990)

Médecine Aromatique, Médecine Planétaire
Vers la fin d'une surveie artificielle (Editions Jollois, 1991)

Pratique Aromatique Familiale (with Rose-Marie Pénoël)
(Editions Osmobiose, 1992)

Urgences et Soins Intensifs en Médecine Aromatique Intégré, Vol. 1 (with Rose-Marie Pénoël) (Editions Osmobiose, 1998)

In preparation:
"The First Aromatic Revolution and the World of the Conifers"
From the Big Bang to the creation of the Aromatic Substance
Vol. I of *Materia Medica* of Integrated Aromatic Medicine

"Rose-Printemps" (CD recording)
Inspired songs composed and interpreted by Rose-Marie Pénoël
(Osmobiose, 1996)

"Method – Rose Printemps" (CD recording)
Accompanied with gemstones and aromatic compositions for each
"energy level" (Chakara)
(Osmobiose, 1997)

TABLE OF CONTENTS

ACKNOWLEDGMENTS
AND
A PLEA FOR GENUINE CIVILITY

"The most mature recorded thinkers have always been mystics and, by definition, systems theorists. One of the constant characteristics of mystics of all cultures and all religions in all ages has been their ever-present consciousness of an invisible interconnectedness beneath the surface of things. Consequently, each of their teachings, one way or another, has de-emphasized the separation between self and other."

M. Scott Peck, MD in "A World Waiting to Be Born," (The Search for Civility), Arrow Press, 1993.

This is the final step in completing the English translation of this book. I have pondered this task for years.

Yesterday, Sunday, June 28, a group of aromatherapists, led by Jim Llewellyn from Melbourne, came to our place for a two hour visit. In the group were members from other parts of Australia (Alexandra from Adelaide who will spend two years in Paris, Sue from Tasmania, Merilyn from Melbourne, and Sue from Sydney), and from other parts of the world (Yvonne from Hong Kong, Naty from Singapore and Mercedes from Cuba, now Florida). It brought a lot of warmth into our hearts to be together and to share our common passion and our vision for the future.

I could not help but think, as I enjoyed the company of these wonderful people from all over the world, that one of the great gifts of aromatic plants and essential oils is to bring together from all over the world, good people who can be wonderful friends. This book, both in its original French and in its new English translation, would not exist without the interconnectedness mentioned in the above quotation.

My function is to be a receiver and a transmitter. To make the message of the Aromatic Revolution available to millions of people throughout the world, I need to be in tune with the rest of the Universe. The feelings I have in my heart are peace, harmony and joy. Another feeling that I want to mention is gratitude. I can only say "thank you" for all that I have received from those with whom I have worked in the past, those I am now working with, and those with whom I will be privileged to work in the future.

I say "thank you" to Mother Nature and to "Gaia," our wonderful planet, the blue pearl of the solar system. Thank you to the plant kingdom and its crown jewels, the aromatic plants with their miraculous creation, namely, tens of thousands of aromatic molecules. Thank you to the entire animal kingdom (especially to the singing birds whose music provides the audio enchantment of our natural environment) for the lessons in humanity its creatures teach us, in particular our close friends, dogs, cats, horses and dolphins. Thank you to Mankind, a full potential of which is still "waiting to be born," but the awakening is starting.

I could fill a book with the names, stories and experiences I have had directly and indirectly through wonderful people connected with natural medicine and essential oils. Let me here identify a few for whom I am especially appreciative.

From the perspective of Aromathérapie, I am grateful to Dr. Jean Valnet, who passed away on the 29th of May, 1995, whose work introduced me to aromathérapie, in the French sense, thirty years ago. I feel a deep connection with René-Maurice Gattefossé, the French chemist who coined the word "aromathérapie" and devoted his life to studying essential oils. R-M Gattefossé died on April 20, 1950, and I was born January 10, 1951. (I was conceived 10 days before his death.) I have felt that my role was to continue the mission he started and develop it further. Among other things, I have been instrumental in researching and launching a new essential oil, which he had tried unsuccessfully to promote during his lifetime. 'Interconnectedness' links us with our predecessors thousands of years ago and extends to all those who continue our research and work after we leave this earth.[1]

I am grateful to my former partner, Pierre Franchomme, with whom I collaborated for thirteen years. The chapter entitled "The Search For Excellence" owes much to his work in botanics and the chemistry of essential oils. He was himself deeply inspired and practically trained by Henri Viaud, to whom I am also highly grateful.

In the context of French-English connections, many friends have played major roles. I have to mention specifically those with whom a close collaboration has taken place:

–Robert Tisserand, who triggered the translation of Dr. Valnet's book into English and edited it. Robert invited me to three great international events, Aroma '93, Aroma '95 and Aroma '97, where I was enabled to present the concepts and applications of Integrated Aromatic Medicine. May he find here the expression of my respect and my encouragement to pursue his worldwide mission, in conjunction with the precious pharmacological research accomplished by Tony Balacs.

–Shirley and Len Price, who realized the importance of going beyond the 'aromatic massage' and organized a special training course for health professionals, especially nurses, in which I have taught Intensive Aromatic Care. Many patients have subsequently received help that was not possible in the traditional aromatherapeutic approach. May they accept my warm thankfulness and my best wishes for the continuation of their dedicated and intense teaching and writing work.

–Valerie Ann Worwood has long been involved in training patients how to help themselves with essential oils and other natural therapies. In this sense, her efforts are similar to ours in creating a natural, aromatic approach to natural home health care. May her charisma and enthusiasm continue to be a source of inspiration and positive action for many people.

–Michael Scholes, from Los Angeles, who played a crucial role in organizing the first training in medical aromatherapy in London (September, 1987) and has trained thousands of students in North America. He made us come several times to the U.S., and he knows the deep and strong link that connects us, through the very special adventures we lived together.

Rose-Marie and I thank him for all that he has done and send him and his partner Joan our friendly thoughts and best wishes to go on "working in and for the Light."

–Kurt Schnaubelt, who played a key role in creating a strong German-French-English connection in aromatherapy. His earnestness and his involvement in high quality products are praiseworthy. May he find here my wishes of ongoing development for his admirable work.

–Marcel Lavabre, a French compatriot, living now in Los Angeles, who brought a great and significant contribution to the development of aromatherapy in North America, and who, along with Kurt Schnaubelt and Victoria Edwards, created the first association in America for aromatherapists. We send him hearty greetings from southern France, which he loves so much and where he was trained in the fine art of distillation. May he pursue his American dream and mission with all the success and reward he deserves.

–John Steele, also from Los Angeles, has always been a source of inspiration, deep reflection and humility by putting things in their proper perspective of archeological time; may he find here our best wishes for a fulfillment of his subtle and highly refined research.

–Peter Holmes, whose integral approach with essential oil potentials is fascinating and brings a remarkable extension to the understanding of healing with aromatic substances. I thank him for his precious contribution in building the "aromatic cathedral."

–Diana Ruzzo, from New York, who has faithfully followed the "osmobiotic discipline" for many years and has experienced such an improvement in her own health that she wrote a comprehensive essay to explain and testify of the efficacy of the whole method.

–Ron Guba in Australia, who played a major role by taking over our mission there, and enabling us to return to Europe with a quiet conscience. He has since been actively involved in the development of clinical and medical aromatherapy throughout Australia and New Zealand. May he accept our warmest wishes for complete success in his research, his teaching and his "live aromatic experiments" on himself.

I have special thoughts for all those who are deeply involved in the production of high quality Tea Tree oil, which is a staple essential oil in aromatic medicine. The following deserve specific mention from me:

–Christopher Dean, with whom we spent Christmas, 1986, and whose contribution has been invaluable both in agricultural development and in commercial distribution of this valuable essential oil.

–Bill McGilvray, helped by his wife, Judith, who has a permanent passion for obtaining the highest quality EOs and who is working very hard to develop new aromatic resources and to establish a reliable system of organic certification for Australian essential oils.

–Prof. Lyall Williams, from Macquarie University, who spent many years studying the chemistry of Tea Tree Oil and ended up getting involved in producing it for therapeutic applications. I want to make special mention to the memory of his assistant, Vicky Home, who passed away in October, 1997. I learned much from all of these Australian producers, from both a scientific and a human point of view. May they accept and receive my feelings of appreciation, which are further extended to all "Aussies" who work so hard to offer the rest of the world the "essence" of their continent in the form of high quality essential oils.

–Judith White and Karen Day, two well-known aromatic sisters from Melbourne, who have shared their love and enthusiasm for essential oils with hundreds of thousands of lay people. I still remember when I asked them to play the role of immune cells, on stage, at Aroma '93 at Brighton University. They did a masterful job of helping me illustrate the concept of aromatic molecules, essential oils and aromatherapy as the "immune system of Mankind." We will meet again when we next visit Australia...

–Bo Hendgen, from New Zealand, land of Manuka and Kanuka, a well-known osteopath in Auckland, who was driven from Germany to New

Zealand (as we were led from France to Australia) by a prophetic dream. I wish her all the best with the implementation of natural and aromatic medicine in conjunction with osteopathy.

–In England, an interesting a medically-oriented work is being accomplished by Rosalind Blackwell, Alan Barker, Maureen Farell and her husband, Vivian Lunny, MD, Gabriel Mojay and many others who received directly or indirectly the French influence. They all know that close links unite us and that we have together succeeded in building an "aromatic Eurotunnel."

–The work and research accomplished by Gabriel Mojay in relationship with Chinese medicine and philosophy and the realm of spiritual healing is a source of great inspiration. Thank you for being such a good and sensitive receiver and transmitter of the "harmonies of the Universe."

–Julia Fisher, Laraine Kyle, Cheryl Hoard, Charla Devereux, Jeanne Rose, Bernie Hephrun, Valerie Cooksley, and countless other herbalists, aromatherapists and natural medicine practitioners, in all English-speaking countries, please accept my thankfulness for your theoretical, practical and organizational work.

–I thank Marianne Denniston (New York) who has developed a wholehearted vision of the planet and its aromatic continents, each bringing the best of their essential oil resources. I wish her the best in the accomplishment of her beautiful dream.

–Sylla Sheppard-Hanger who has brought an encompassing contribution to the understanding of aromatic molecules, essential oils and their many actions. May she find here my congratulations for her intense on-going work and my support for the continuation of her important task

–Galina Lisin, who is animated by a passion for the highest quality aromatic products and displays a strong "Russian will" to establish high training standards in America.

–In Germany, my friend Martin Henglein who opened for me a new way of understanding the subtle aspect of essential oils and "forced" me to return to the German language in order to present, with great success, Integral Aromatherapy and Integrated Aromatic Medicine to German-speaking aromatherapists.

–In Israel, Mr. Haim Schloss who organized the first training in Integrated Aromatic Medicine in Tel Aviv in 1997, helped by Julie Loven who courageously translated my English lectures into Hebrew. Rosy Abelsohn, from Jerusalem University, specialist in immunology, who now has a true love affair with aromatherapy and essential oils. Her collaboration will be valuable for the scientific and medical development of aromatherapy in this "from the first days blessed" country.

–In Norway Gry Fossvedt, who organized the first seminar in Oslo in April, 1995, for Integral Aromatherapy and Integrated Aromatic Medicine. I wish her great success with her new book, for which I wrote the forward.

–In Japan, Mr. Isao Tsunoda (Tokyo), who organized our venue in his country and made my teaching available to Japanese aromatherapists.

For my medical training, I thank my professors at the Paris Medical University (connected with Saint Antoine Hospital). For my training in natural medicine, I thank all the great naturopaths from all over the world whose influence shaped my thinking in medicine and integral aromatherapy. For my training in homeopathy, I thank all my teachers in France. For my training is auriculotherapy, I thank Drs. Nogier, Bourdiol and Kovacs. For my training in energy medicine and chromatotherapy, I thank Dr. Christian Agrapart who opened to my mind a new field of understand, with exciting clinical applications.

Above all, I thank my patients from all over the world, especially Abby, from whom I have learned so much. From a psychological point of view, my deep thanks are sent to all the renown psychologists in all English-speaking countries whose books have brought a revolution in this field similar to the one that is occurring in medicine with essential oils and aromatherapy. Particularly I feel indebted toward Dr. Wayne Dyer for his writings and teachings. What I am living now is exactly in tune with what he teaches about a "sense of mission to be accomplished." It is at the core of my way of thinking and acting. I know we will meet one day.

–Special thanks to my dear wife, Rose-Marie, who has been totally involved in the "aromatic passion," sometimes with much struggle and difficulty, and also our three children, who have not seen their father as much as they should have, because he was completely absorbed in aromatic adventures.

Concerning more specifically this book, I thank Dr. Gary Young, his wife, Mary, and their team of workers for their unfailing support and for making possible its publication in conjunction with my return to the U.S. in July, 1998. I congratulate Gary for his incredible agricultural and distillation accomplishments in Utah and Idaho. This is precisely my picture of 'healing the planet' and creating a vast, beautiful and fragrant garden. His permanent collaboration with French growers and distillers creates a strong link starting from the earth and from the world of plants themselves. May he find here my deep wishes for the beginning of a new unification process in North American aromatherapy.

I thank all those who have worked so hard to translate my French way of thinking and expressing myself into readable American English, namely, Daniel Belgique and his team of translators in the U.S., and Christopher Wessel and Laurence Delatour in France. I thank the team at Bailey-Montague & Associates, particularly Paul Springer and Robin Sheppick, who completed the layout and typesetting under very tight and sometimes frustrating deadlines. Also, my thanks go to Mark Burdge and his staff at Excel Graphics, who found a way to print the book in just five working days so it would be available at the Salt Lake Seminar. And I send special thoughts of deep gratitude to Brian Manwaring who worked as the chief editor almost 24 hours a day on this project. We share a philosophy of making things happen. As Wayne Dyer puts it, "we will see it when we believe it." May he find here the expression of my joy to have found, in addition to a valuable collaborator, a true friend, which is not so common these days.

Many others are earnestly working for spread of aromatherapy and the use of essential oils in medical applications. I feel fully and deeply interconnected with all of them. They comprise a true "spiritual Internet" that can work without electricity or computers!

I know perfectly well that there are many others who deserve mention here but time and space will not allow it. I include them in my collective thoughts of gratitude and appreciation on the occasion of the publication of my first English language book.

As a final note, and not necessarily a happy one, I have found, traveling all over the world, that contentious relationships exist between some individuals and groups involved in aromatherapy. This is not confined to a single state, a single country or a single continent, but is a worldwide weakness that prevents a more rapid acceptance of aromatic medicine. Even among the wonderful people named above there exist divisions and dissensions that are unbecoming of a gift so great as essential oils. These internal conflicts have often been the source of deep sadness for me, and I feel compelled to do all I can to eliminate them. So I have chosen to write a little extension to this acknowledgments section, directed not so much to the new student in aromatherapy, but rather to those who are in positions of influence to create harmony. I call the section that follows "a plea for genuine civility" and ask for your understanding and patience in reading it. I understand this is an unusual approach, but I am "above-guided" to do it this way, lest it will not be "above-permitted" for this book to be successfully released in the world markets.

A PLEA FOR
GENUINE CIVILITY

A lay person, or one new to the science and art of aroma-therapy might not be directly concerned about–or even aware of–the fierce competition that exists between individuals, firms, teaching institutes and training schools involved in the industry. The fact that it does exist has always been appalling to me. It seems like such crude behavior for people involved with some of nature's most refined and complex substances. It is a disease, and no essential oil has the power to "cure" it. The cure must come from deep inside the heart.

I would like to share some personal observations and feelings on this subject, but what I am about to say applies in all areas of life, be they personal or professional. After all, we cannot really expect our professional conduct to be materially different than our personal conduct.

There is a forgiveness process involved in acquiring a genuine civility. Human graciousness is impossible without it. And it must be understood in order to read this book in an ideal state of openness, humility and desire for truth, which will lead to a lasting personal transformation.

The best way I can describe my feelings about struggles for power and control (financially, politically or intellectually) is by comparing them with the surface of the sea, agitated by wind and waves. When we dive deeply below the surface, we find a world of ultimate quietness, tranquility and peace. The interconnectedness beneath the surface of human relations is an incontrovertible reality, whether we accept it or not.

Let me first tell you a story. It is a true story, a sad story, that took place in the highest medical circles of France:

> Those familiar with Chinese traditional acupuncture might have heard of Georges Soulié de Morand. He was a long-time ambassador of France in China. Although not educated as a doctor, he had the opportunity to study the philosophy and practice of Chinese medicine and acupuncture. He had a tremendous passion for the subject and learned it well. He was, of course, a diplomat, not a doctor, but he recognized the priceless value in acupuncture and wanted to bring it back to France. When he returned from his diplomatic post, he began training medical doctors in this new science. Many French doctors got their first insights into acupuncture from this skilled man. Once his MD "pupils" had obtained from him whatever they could get, they decided to sue him in front of the Medical Board (the equivalent of the AMA in the U.S.) for illegally practicing medicine. The reason was not difficult to discern. Recognizing that there was a powerful new modality now in the hands of a non-doctor, they needed to remove the threat of losing face…and money…from someone outside their "club."

We see stories like this reproduced like a permanent and universal pattern in almost every field of human activity. One would have hoped that somehow in aromatherapy, where we deal with the quintessence of harmony, things might have been different. Unfortunately, that does not yet seem to be the case. Much of the problem arises from not respecting each other's efforts.

There are three basic ways we abuse someone else's work.

1. A person simply uses information provided by someone else and is naive and insensitive to the importance of giving proper credit to the original source. It is an error of omission, but there is no malevolent intent.

2. A person obtains insight or information from another and, seeking to claim it as his own, refuses to acknowledge the real source of the information. It is a deliberate act. It is a serious offense, demonstrating a complete lack of respect and civility. It is a form of stealing and those who engage in it suffer all their lives from a subconscious guilt that, like a thorn in a shoe, hurts at every step of life.

3. Person A obtains insight or information from Person B, but in this case, although A would like to claim it as his own, it is well-known that this knowledge originated with B. The only course left to A is a destructive one–trying to discredit or slander the work/information/skills that B developed, so B may no longer derive benefit therefrom. This is an even more serious offense. And guess what? The Book of Books–both in the Old and New Testaments–fully describes and analyzes these same behaviors.

This attitude of "killing the father" (the word "father" here being interpreted in a broad sense, i.e. author, teacher, healer, etc.) is described in a French expression as "le pain de la honte" (the bread of shame). A person or group receives "bread," meaning anything good, and they feel within, consciously or subconsciously, that they are not worthy of this very special good gift. Instead of trying to improve so that they will eventually deserve this gift, they find it easier to turn against the author or provider of the gift and try to destroy him in one way or another. I have seen many situations like this in the world of medicine in general, and–even more unfortunately, in the world of natural medicine.

Dear reader, let me make one very important observation: all those I have known who have engaged in this type of criminal conduct, have ended their careers–sometimes even their lives– in a miserable condition. This is the well-known "boomerang effect." Part of my purpose is to establish more respect, greater harmony and fair, real, recognized civility.

Envy, jealousy, anger and pride are behind contention. They form a disease that can be cured. (Those who become addicted to it and cultivate it, will reap the harvest they deserve.) To help those who want help in being cured from it, I submit the following three mental screenplays. I encourage you to read and ponder carefully the dynamics inherent in this simple situations

Think of the person you feel is your worst enemy. Maybe you have never even met him or her personally, but you have heard so many bad things about this person that you are sure he or she deserves to be destroyed in one way or another. Now consider the following:

Screenplay Number 1:

Imagine that this enemy is a victim, let's say, in a car accident on an isolated road and you happen to drive past the scene. You stop and recognize your enemy, injured and bleeding. He/she is not conscious, but still alive. There is no one else around.

Would you withdraw quickly, leaving your enemy to die? Nobody would ever know that you could have saved his/her life, but did not because of the malice in your heart. Or would you have saved this enemy anyway, no matter what you believe or have been led to believe about this person?

Screenplay Number 2:

Now, it is the reverse situation. You are the one in the accident on a remote road; but this time, you are still conscious. Your enemy drives past your car smashed against a tree. He stops his car. Perhaps he does not even know you, but you recognize him immediately. Would you refuse to let him help you and save your life? Remember, it is an isolated road and no other car will drive on it in time to save your life. Perhaps you think to yourself: He is such a bad person that he will never do anything good for me or for anyone else. But to your surprise, he immediately calls the paramedics on his cell phone and puts his whole love and care into providing emergency first aid while waiting for the rescue team. Don't you think you would begin to ponder more seriously the negative gossip or rumor you had heard about this enemy? Owing your very life to his concerned and helpful intervention, do you believe you will go on cultivating the same negative attitudes toward him and nurturing the same bad feelings, which in reality are destructive only to yourself?

Screenplay Number 3:

This time, the scenario takes place in the mountains and it happens that you find yourself in a difficult situation together with your enemy. Each of you and both of you can only be saved if each of you and both of you agree to work together and help one another. If one refuses, both of you will perish! Would you refuse? Can you imagine for one second that such an incredibly stupid thing is possible? Personally, I can't. If you think you might refuse, do you know who your worst enemy really is? Yourself, of course. And isn't it the case, most of the time, that when you think of anyone as an enemy and emit thoughts of aggression or animosity, you do become your worst enemy.

Imagining hypothetically extreme situations, as in the above "screen-plays." is a mental activity which is quite common in physics and even more so in mathematics. It is an exercise that can be extremely useful in understanding less extreme situations. If you really projected seriously as you read these screenplays; if you really went through the mental pictures, I feel certain you will have had new thoughts about your so-called enemy. Perhaps you will have broken a barrier of prejudice. Perhaps you will have seen some of your own faults in greater clarity. If you have succeeded, even a little bit, in changing old and distorted opinions for better and healthier ones, it is worth far more than the price you paid for this book. You can apply this exercise of extreme situations with all your imagined enemies. If you do it properly and sincerely in a silent, private place, making the mental pictures as vivid to your mind as you can, I am sure you will soon become a new person. It will be a person that is more like the 'real' you. And you will have gained new freedom of thought and feeling. You will feel lighter and relieved. You will probably sense a tiny bit of the interconnectedness and tranquility that lies below the surface of human interaction. You will begin to see things happening in your life that you never thought possible before. Please do it; and give me your feedback.

Now, the truth is that extreme situations exist right now; and we are all in the same boat. Cutthroat competition is deadly! What we need is support and cooperation; complete symbiosis between those of us who share the same values. Finding ways to regain and rebuild a genuine civility among us, should be our permanent goal. This is the core of Dr. Speck's wonderful book. If we do not succeed in this noble task, our world will continue down the path of self-destructive craziness. My heart of hearts tells me that–at least in the world of aromatherapy–there are more people who want peace, fruitful exchange and cooperation than there are who want constant struggle and interpersonal war. What kind of feeling motivates the contention among us? What is the root cause? Any ideas?

You might say it is the sin of pride or arrogance that triggers the situation? Or perhaps selfishness and greed? I think we need to look deeper. I believe the root cause is fear; more specifically fear of being without. Being without success, money, recognition, admiration, knowledge, power, influence, etc. This is one of the worst fears of all; one that can lead to permanent personal and social dysfunction.

The best advice I can give to counteract and eliminate this fear is to trust yourself. Trust your true self, not the selfish or greedy or power-hungry self. Trust the self that is deep inside, in the quiet and tranquility way below the stormy surface. Trust the Universe. Trust that the great Creator has built a world that will provide you with what you need to give the best of yourself during your sojourn here on planet Earth.

Because I am almost certain you love music, I will end this plea for civility with another true story. This one has a happier ending.

You probably have enjoyed the great music of Ludwig von Beethoven. I share a great appreciation for his creative genius. But there is someone else who felt this deep admiration to a point that it became a stumbling block for him. I'm sure his name is familiar to you. He was Johannes Brahms. The intensity of Brahms' admiration for Beethoven was so great that he felt he would never be able to compose music on the same level as Beethoven. This feeling created a mental paralysis within Brahms. It stopped him rather than inspired him. As this mental block grew, Brahms began to have more and more difficulty composing good music. Finally, he reached a mental crisis. He could choose to forget the intimidation he felt and compose the best that was within him, or he could continue to be paralyzed by his fear that he was not on the same level as his idol. Thank God, Brahms was able to decide to go forward, and once past this mental block, he created some of the richest music we know today. It was not like Beethoven's, but it was still wonderful.

It has been said that "most men die with their music still in them." That cannot be said of Brahms. Let it not be said of you or of me. Open your mind to Truth, devote your heart to Beauty, dedicate your soul to Good and let your spirit operate according to Right. You will then be able to release the 'music' that is in the real you. You will become the creator of the most beautiful work of art you could ever imagine: your own life!

Enjoy your reading, and I'll meet you personally at the end of the book to welcome you to a profound and holistic transformation.

Dr. Daniel Pénoël, Drôme Valley, June 30, 1998.

FOREWORD
by Abby Bean
Adelaide, Australia

nhampered by sickness now, I find it hard to recall the years of my life when illness played a major role. From birth until the age of seven, I was never truly healthy. In old photos, I appear pale and skinny, often with my mouth open to facilitate breathing because of an almost constantly blocked nose. The complete metamorphosis I have experienced, from the sickly child I was at seven to the robust person I am now, did not occur overnight.

I lived daily with the effects of my illnesses before meeting Dr. Pénoël. Sickness was for me a way of life. Now, my memories of this trying time are hazy and I can only reconstruct an abstract view of my poor health when compared to my present health. I compiled the following story through a number of different view points: those of my parents and relatives, the medical reports I have read, and the scattered shreds of my own memory...

Once there was a little girl who was sick for a very long time. Sore ears and a snotty nose were not an unusual state of affairs for her. Her teeth had become rotten as the drugs she took to get well slowly destroyed her resistance to infection. Her knees and stomach were so painful at times that she screamed in pain. This child was me.

From the age of two months it became apparent that I was not going to be a healthy child. Born in 1979, two weeks premature, I spent my first days in a humidicrib. A series of infections followed and between the years 1981 and 1983, my doctors administered thirty separate courses of antibiotics, prescribed to cure me of various infections. What the antibiotics actually achieved was the gradual breakdown of my resistance to illness and infection.

By the age of seven I had suffered many bouts with flu, tonsillitis, ear infections, and common colds. The antibiotics I took did little to improve my overall health. My nose was always running. I suffered earaches and pains in my legs and stomach. I had little energy. As a result of inner ear infections, I had poor balance and often had grazes on my knees. Besides all this, my teeth were weakened from prolonged use of antibiotics and my mouth was full of fillings. As I read this list, I am amazed that my memories are not more horrific or rueful, yet I must restate that this was a way of life for me, a day-to-day existence. I simply did not know what it was like to be healthy, and could only envy my healthy and active friends.

Although I now remember little of this time, I do recall the general feeling of taking an endless array of necessary precautions. Friends of the family who had colds were not allowed to come to visit. My breakfast was always accompanied with vitamin tablets and often antibiotics. I was unable to eat milk or wheat products because of my allergies. I underwent three separate operations for the insertion and reinsertion of grommets in my ears to prevent further ear infections (a painful and terrorizing experience for a young child). Because of these operations I had to wear earplugs when swimming or even in the shower. My family and I accepted this way of life, but kept looking for alternatives, aware that my body would eventually become used to the antibiotics I was taking and would need larger doses. The antibiotics were weakening my immune system, and as I got weaker, I needed more antibiotics to keep me well. I was caught in a vicious cycle from which my family and I saw no escape.

The events that led up to my discovery of aromatherapy and a pathway to health all started in 1986 when, after a prolonged and serious bout of ear infections and sinus pain, I was again referred to an ENT specialist.

After x-rays were taken, the specialist informed my parents that the build-up of puss in my sinuses could only be corrected through a scraping operation under general anaesthesia. At this point my parents were really beginning to question the effectiveness of conventional medicine. As there was no guarantee that this operation would prevent a similar build-up in the future, we hesitated. Together, we made the decision that I would not have the operation. As a family, we had discussed the alternatives. Having heard of a French doctor, a GP who was also a naturopath and had recently arrived in Adelaide, we sought his advice over the phone. After that call, we informed the specialist that we had decided to pursue other methods for clearing up my condition. He told us that such actions would be taken at "your own risk" and that he wished me to have another x-ray and appointment with him in two weeks.

The first appointment with Dr. Daniel Pénoël produced mixed reactions in me. Although I was always a shy child, his accent intrigued me and his office was an amazing and mysterious place. The natural scent of eucalyptus and rosemary and other essential oils was not at all like the smell of disinfectant to which I had become accustomed. The strange and twisted paraphernalia that lined his walls captured my curious attention from the moment I entered the door. It was like an adventure when compared with other doctors' offices which I, by then, knew too well.

Over the next two weeks I had appointments with Dr. Pénoël eleven times. By the end of that time, the amazement had worn off and, like all small children, I had become tired of the discipline and routine involved. However, the intense and sometimes fantastic treatments I received there and continued in my own home were not undertaken fruitlessly. Those two weeks of trials and tribulations were to change my life forever.

The first changes happened promptly and drastically after that first appointment. Dr. Pénoël and his wife Rose-Marie worked with me and my parents, instructing us on how to continue at home the intensive treatments and keep up the new diet I had received. In this way my family and I were offered a way to take control of my health so that we would be almost self-sufficient in the future.

My diet, already lacking milk and wheat products, was to suffer the further loss of peanut butter (my favourite spread for toast), bananas, apple skin, egg whites, and much more. In addition, I was required to eat, drink, and breathe essential oils. I was almost bathed in their heady, intense aromas for twenty-four hours each day. Before bed I was massaged with them; during the night I breathed them in through an amazing array of twisted and blown glass aerosol equipment. I sprayed my throat with a rosemary oil mixture and swallowed essential oils mixed with honey. At night the beautiful aromas of the essential oils, were somewhat diluted by the sauteed onions which encased my feet!

Most of these treatments occurred at home under the instruction of Dr.
Pénoël. However, other strange and wonderful procedures went on during
the office appointments I attended almost every day after school. Magnets
were attached behind my ears and knees (a treatment which made my
parents a little skeptical) and Dr. Pénoël conducted a painless laser treatment on some parts of my body, feet, and face. Strange electrical magnetic
paddles were applied to my cheeks which were also massaged with other
equipment. I was instructed to sit still and, trial of all trials, not to talk while
I breathed in a strong mixture of oil vapours. During this time, in between
the long and sometimes arduous treatments, Dr. Pénoël's children were
often present, offering me their support and friendship when I would
otherwise have felt awkward and lonely.

If I had had any idea of the outcome of these treatments, I would have
begged for more. However, I was not used to the self-discipline and end-
lessly complicated and taxing routines necessary to ensure a swift cleansing
of my system. Familiar only with the relatively effortless prescriptions of
antibiotics, I complained long and loud. Unlike the antibiotics I was used
to, these intense treatments required personal input and effort from me
and each of my family members. Without my parents' dedication to these
new routines and the Pénoël family's kind and unflagging support and
attention, it would have been almost impossible to bear.

After two weeks I went back for the second x-ray. What conventional
medicine had been trying to do for seven years was essentially done in
two weeks. My condition was cleared. The x-ray showed no need for an
operation!

The ENT specialist said these "unexplainable" and "spontaneous" recov-
eries were known to occur at times in children. He could not believe that
any medicine other than his own could be so effective. Aromatherapy had
won the first battle in my fight for health. However, the struggle along the
road to overall health had just started.

This miraculous and swift recovery from an infection which conventional doctors believed could only be cured through an operation, proved
to be only the tip of the iceberg. Dr. Pénoël started us on a road toward
the ultimate goal which I am now able to enjoy.

In July, 1986, I again became ill with a brown mucus discharge being
found on my pillow each morning. Dr. Pénoël, who was contacted at a

medical conference where he was lecturing in Melbourne, assured my parents that this was yet another stage in my full recovery. They were worried that they could not lower my soaring temperatures with conventional medicines. Dr. Pénoël gave detailed instructions over the phone.

His work in conjunction with my family, more as a tutor than a doctor, teaching my parents and I what must be done each day and night, which oils were effective for which symptoms, etc., enabled my parents to continue my care during times when he was not available. Imagine our mutual joy when, after returning from Melbourne, he found me almost fully recovered.

For me, these two astounding developments in my treatment and recovery are not as memorable as an incident which occurred two years later. After two years of sticking to the strict diet, daily massage, and essential oils which had gradually restored my health to that of normal, rebellious nine-year old, I decided to go off my diet.

Every day on the way to school, my friends and I stopped at a deli where they purchased rich cream buns. The next ten minutes were filled with the rapturous moans of my companions as they ate these delicacies, in which I had never been able to indulge. The temptation finally proved too much. Reasoning that I had been healthy all year, I bought one. Filled with rich cream, the wheat flour bun was coated with chocolate icing almost a centimetre thick! I devoured it!...and then waited for the inevitable sinus attack.

Two years earlier, this one bun would have had my nose streaming and my chest sore with coughing for weeks. I expected the worst...but nothing happened! After two years of continued use of alternative medicine, I remained well (despite the guilt).

Alternative medicine had not weakened my immune system as conventional medicine had. It had not worked merely as a preventative medicine but had improved my overall well-being and strengthened my body against infection. Alternative medicine continued to triumph over my previous illnesses and I was able to gradually broaden my diet.

Now, at seventeen, I am a robust teenager. I love cold weather and the exhilaration of brisk walks across the hills of my university campus. I rarely get sick and usually do not catch the common colds to which I am exposed. I always turn first to alternative medicine and aromatherapy to get rid of colds. I feel very lucky to have discovered alternative medicine. I shudder to think what my life would have been like without the strength given to me through the healing influence of essential oils, effective natural processes, and the dedicated and compassionate help of Dr. Daniel Pénoël and his family and mine.

Through alternative medicine I have been able to achieve the healthy lifestyle that was once only a dream. I can only hope that, in the future, the alternative medicines which changed my life will be readily available to all, and that the essences of nature will be recognised by all doctors as effective treatments for disease and illness.

Abby Bean
Adelaide, South Australia
May 16, 1996

AUTHOR'S PREFACE TO THE ENGLISH EDITION

Aouste-sur Sye
Vallée de la Drôme
France
May 31, 1998

Dear reader,

*T*his book was written and published in 1992 in its original French version. It is with great joy that I welcome its translation into the English language. This joy is all the more intense since the central history of little Abby Bean–New Zealand-born and Australian-raised–perfectly symbolizes the potential of a French-English connection in using essential oils to re-establish, maintain and improve human health.

How did it happen that a French doctor, successful in his practice of natural and aromatic medicine in his own country, decided to 'leave it all behind' and take his wife and three children on an adventure to the Australian continent? The answer is the subject of another future book, the story behind this story. For now, let me simply certify to you that my commitment to aromatic medicine has not only sustained me, but also guided me and my family through hundreds of extraordinary adventures of a truly planetary dimension.[2]

Millions of lives have been, are, and will be transformed thanks to the judicious and regular use of the precious life substances extracted from aromatic plants: the essential oils. Playing a key role in globalizing high quality aromatherapy as a doctor, teacher, speaker, researcher and writer has been the great satisfaction of my career.

Our Australian experience was an indispensable element in the fulfillment of my life's mission, namely, to establish a method of health care crucial for the coming century. For a Frenchman to embark on an international medical career requires some intimate experience and association with the English-speaking world. Australia, with its immense aromatic resources, was an incredible opportunity for me to develop my English abilities and at the same time become immersed in the land of the eucalyptus and the melaleucas.

Twelve years have passed since the initial phase (1986) of Abby's healing, described in her foreword for this book. During those twelve years, we have seen a tremendous increase in the dissemination of aromatherapeutic medical information from France to the rest of the world, beginning with the Anglo-Saxon countries. With this foundation, medical aromatherapy will advance now at an ever-increasing pace.

The days when new alternatives were viewed as an "underground" science, as described by American journalist Marilyn Ferguson in her "Aquarian Conspiracy" of the 1980's, are now fully past. The dawn of a new century is upon us. We are living on the face of a planet which has become as interconnected and as interdependent as a small village. Humanity and the Biosphere are at a crossroads. To refuse any longer to embrace truth, to ignore the peril of our world and to continue our irresponsible commercial behaviors at the planet's expense, constitutes an attitude that is indolent, unworthy and morally unacceptable.

On the 21st and 22nd of March, 1998, the First International Symposium of Integrated Aromatic Medicine was held in the city of Grasse, France. I was the instigator and the planner for this extremely successful symposium. Additionally, I served as the president of the medical-scientific committee. On the occasion of this event, I released the first volume of a new collection entitled "Introduction to Integrated Aromatic Medicine."[3]

Initially, we had planned to have this volume translated to English to mark my return to the U.S. (after seven years dedicated to the rest of the world), exactly four months after the Grasse Symposium. On July 21st and 22nd, I will present a two-day training seminar on Integrated Aromatic Medicine in Salt Lake City, Utah, at the invitation of Dr. Gary Young. Dr. R. Young himself attended the Grasse Symposium and made a three-part presentation there, including his landmark work in the areas of organic farming and steam distilling for U.S. production of therapeutic grade essential oils.

But both because of lack of time and to preserve a sense of logical development and progression, the decision was made to translate and publish this book, instead. Part I of the book deals primarily with theory and philosophy and has not been changed. Part II, however, which focuses on the practical applications involved in home health care with essential oils, has been reworked, adapted and updated to reflect more current research and practice.

My primary goal is first and foremost to educate, to inform. I want to build sufficient understanding in the minds of my readers that they will be motivated to begin the task of daily self-management, using the principles of this book, to create vibrant health for every family unit.

In order to aid the English-speaking public in understanding the concept of aromatherapy in its clinical, medical and pharmaceutical context, I feel it worthwhile to outline the historic development of the French approach to aromatherapy and contrast it with the English approach. Historically and fundamentally these two approaches are different, though complimentary.

The triad of primary aromatic orientations

The word "aromatherapy" has today become a household word, not only in the English-speaking countries, but all over the surface of the planet. But this word, in fact, is used to refer to realities and practices which are completely different, depending on one's cultural orientation. If one can understand the nature of aromatic plants and essential oils on three levels, namely as Matter, Energy and Information, then one can easily comprehend the reasons for these semantic differences.

In my instruction, I illustrate aromatherapy differences with a three-sided triangle. Each point is represented by a language-based culture, i.e., French-speaking cultures (France, Belgium, Switzerland, Quebec) represent one point; German-speaking cultures (unified Germany, Austria, Switzerland) represent a second point and English-speaking cultures (British Isles, North America, Australia, etc.) the third point. We thus end up with three points labeled with three consecutive letters of the alphabet: E, F, and G, representing English, French and German.

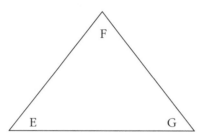

This triangle clearly illustrates the three great orientations to the practice of aromatherapy.[4] In what I call English Style Aromatherapy (ESA), the image that comes to mind is that of a person receiving a relaxing and health-promoting full-body aromatic massage with essential oils diluted in a base of vegetable oil. This model corresponds to an attitude well-expressed by the verb "caring" in its most noble and profound sense.[5] Aromatic massage is a true gift of self which is given to the person being cared for.

The approach that developed in German-speaking cultures places primary emphasis on the aspect of "duft" (scent or fragrance), and inhaling that fragrance. When one compares the deep and intimate feelings evoked by beautiful music with the impressions and vibrations evoked by aromatic sensations, one can see that a very real analogy exists between these two sensory perceptions. Now, which countries have given the world the greatest number of composers and musical geniuses? Obviously, Germany and Austria, two German-speaking countries. I do not wish to imply that the fragrance and olfactory perception aspects of essential oils have been ignored by other cultures; my international exposure simply leads me to observe that this aspect receives more emphasis from the German cultures. Having the good fortune and happiness of sincere friendships and coop-eration with the German-speaking world of aromatherapy, I developed an appreciation for their passionate approach to the olfactory aspects of essential oils.[6]

As for my native country, if you ask what best symbolizes France in the eyes of the rest of the world, there is unanimous agreement. France presents itself above all as the country of eating well and drinking well. It is a country of gastronomy, especially in cheeses, but also wines and spirits, the products of vineyards rich in a tradition of love and tender care for the soil, plants and animals that live thereon. France, which is characterized by the important place of "orality" in its culture, is the same country which has developed a particular emphasis on the oral use of aromatic extracts (including the use of numerous aromatic prescriptions that enter by way of the "other end" of the digestive tract...in the form of suppositories or diluted aromatic rectal injections).

In fact, the word "aromathérapie" as used in the French language, does not mean the same thing as the word "aromatherapy" as used in the UK. How did this different reality come about on opposite sides of the English Channel? I will explain through a historical and geographical analysis of events that occurred in the twentieth century.

The birth and initial development of aromatherapy in France

Aromatic plants have been the object of respect and veneration among the majority of civilizations of the past. Their extracts have been used to provide health to the body, elevation to the soul, relief to the spirit, and also for beauty, cooking, preventative care and healing. I want to focus particularly on the recent history of aromatherapy, especially its 'official' birth in France.

The word "aromatherapy" was invented, coined, by the chemist René-Maurice Gattefossé in Lyon in the 1930's. He worked in close cooperation with doctors, pharmacists and surgeons. The point of departure for development of modern aromatherapy in France was therefore primarily within the medical and pharmaceutical communities. Another name now well-known, is that of Dr. Jean Valnet, whose career was dedicated to natural medicine and the use of phyto-aromatherapy.[7] Today France counts hundreds of doctors and pharmacists who have been trained in phyto-aromatherapy and who are enthusiastic about the medical use of plants in various forms. Given the strength of action and the concentration of essential oils, it is normal that they should be the object of specialized study and practice.

Aromatic medicine is recognized in France as being so important and so effective that it has been established as a medical specialty. When someone from France or a French-speaking country says he is undergoing an aromatherapy treatment, he is talking about serious medical therapy. Following an initial consultation, he has received a specific prescription from a doctor trained in medical aromatherapy and has gone to a specialized pharmacy to obtain different preparations for use: drops, gelcaps, syrups, suppositories, preparations for external application, essential oil blends for inhalation, for aerosols, for baths or for compresses, etc.

By contrast, when someone from England says he is undergoing an aromatherapy treatment, he is talking about a relaxing session of body massage with diluted essential oils (ESA). This concept of aromatherapy is practically unknown in France. Moreover, the profession of aromatherapist does not exist in and of itself, and there are currently no French institutions which train and certify individuals as ESA-type aromatherapists.

Efforts which brought a scientific research approach to natural medical aromatherapy actually did not begin in earnest until the middle of the 1970's, making medical aromatherapy one of the newest specialties in medicine today.

In the 1930's, when R-M Gattefossé was doing his research, aromatic plants were not chemically cultivated. But chemically-oriented agro-business began to spread at great speed following World War II. By 1950 chemical pollution of the soil and plants was so widespread that it was difficult to claim one was caring for people "naturally," knowing that most of the plants used for treatment were gorged with pesticides. This concern motivated a number of distillers to orient themselves back to a truly organic production of essential oils and floral waters, so they could offer full guarantees for therapists and their patients.

Two other important quality issues have been recognized in the past 20 years. First was the need for botanical precision with the plants being distilled. There is tremendous variety among the aromatic species, and although two plants may appear to be the same, there can be significant differences in the principle constituents of their essential oils. Second, was the need for special forms of distillation. Distillation for therapeutic grade essential oils must demonstrate an infinitely greater respect for the plant than is common in the production of essential oils for the perfume, cosmetics or food industries.

After completing my studies at the University of Paris, I had the good fortune to find myself directly involved in the renovation of medical aromatherapy. I was able to participate in the pioneering work dealing with the highest grade essential oils for therapy. For seven years, from 1977 to 1984, I built my private medical practice (in the Paris vicinity) on medical aromatherapy. The clinical, theoretical, technical and practical fundamentals of the methods which I now teach had their origins during this intense period which was rich in discovering new applications for numerous maladies.

(To further help you understand the situation in France, I should clarify that up until December, 1990, all phyto-aromatic prescriptions filled by pharmacists were reimbursed by the government health care system. This greatly facilitated the care of all ill persons, even those who were less well-off financially. The government tried to eliminate this benefit, but the pharmacists fought it and won a technical victory. Today, however, the policy is determined on a county-by-county basis, with some counties allowing the benefit while others do not. Costs for these prescriptions are, of course, much lower than they would be for conventional medical care, especially when it involves people being sent to the hospital.)

My partner, Pierre Franchomme, and I collaborated together on some ground-breaking research which helped us discover many new natural clinical applications. Pierre did the botanical and biochemical research while I was involved in the clinical applications, the practical use and technical development. I had occasion to treat a very wide diversity of diseases in patients of all ages. From the most dramatically acute cases to the most desperately chronic ones, therapeutic grade essential oils played a crucial role in providing significant relief, or in many cases, a total cure. These experiences give me the right and the duty to affirm that when highest quality essential oils are used for therapy, the results are often spectacular–even in cases where all other methods have failed. This has lead me to compare medical aromatherapy to the spearhead of natural medicine. I feel that the highly concentrated nature of essential oils gives them unequaled natural power to transfer life and energy and is the explanation for healings that are sometimes considered miracles.

When a patient, who has been suffering for years in spite of scientific medical care, suddenly sees a significant improvement in a relatively short time, it is understandable that he or she might talk of a "miracle." It is, however, logical and according to research. It is the result of very effective natural medications with complex aromatic molecules that have healing powers not found in synthetic drugs.

The French-English connection in the development of scientific and medical aromatherapy

Through pioneers such as Mrs. Marguerite Maury, essential oil therapy crossed the English Channel and grew in England mainly according to an aspect I call "soft" (or Yin). This approach was widely embraced by beauty therapists in a context of massage and/or spa treatment. Starting from this point, the system of body massage with various diluted essential oils has been applied outside the French-speaking world. It is this 'soft' system that is known and recognized as the principle form of aromatherapy in English-speaking countries.

The first bridges between the English (soft/Yin) and French (hard/Yang) systems of aromatherapy were built both between France and England and between France and Australia. Some are not aware of the important developments in Australia in this respect. Here, it is important to make two observations:

1. France and Australia have in common an abundance of plants that create therapeutic essential oils. They have been blessed by the aromatic gods because of the richness of their flora.

2. During the same period when R-M Gattefossé was doing his analytical work to identify the constituents of essential oils, two Australian scholars, A. R. Penfold and F. R. Morrison, were continuing studies on eucalyptus oils that were already far advanced. This research brought them to the discovery of the existence of chemotypes or chemical races within the same species.

The work I was involved in during my two years in Australia–first in Adelaide, South Australia and then in Melbourne, Victoria–was the equivalent of crossing the first bridge toward developing the French-style medical aromatherapy in an English-speaking country.

An important connection was also being established between France and the United States. Kurt Schnaubelt, a young German chemist, who was passionate about essential oils, chose to emigrate to California at the same time we were receiving our permanent visas to emigrate to Australia. Kurt Schnaubelt had followed the scientific/medical style of aromatherapy provided in France and decided to carry it to the West Coast of the U.S., establishing himself near San Francisco. By curious coincidence (I personally believe that the Universe has a global plan and a mission for each of us) a young American trained by Schnaubelt, Ron Guba, was about to marry an Australian and emigrate to Australia. He played an important role in our decision to leave Adelaide and set ourselves up in Melbourne. He is also the one who took up our activities after we left, and played a key role in the development of clinical/medical aromatherapy in Australia and also New Zealand.

Another Frenchman who played an important role in the development of high quality aromatherapy in North America is Marcel Lavabre, who now lives and trains in the Los Angeles area. Trained at the Provencal School of Distillation[8] in obtaining highest quality aromatic materials, he has contributed much to the progression of the aromatherapy movement in the U.S., through his knowledge and know-how.

In February, 1987, our entire family returned to France. Just five months later an event occurred which I believe was pivotal in building the Franco-English aromatherapy connection, this time in England itself. Pierre Franchomme and I had arranged for a small booth at a large health exhibition and fair in London. A young Englishman, Michael Scholes, was drawn to our booth like a magnet, and practically never left it during that exhibition. At the end of the fair, he knew clearly what his role would be. He perceived his mission with great clarity. He had firmly decided to organize the first training seminar for scientific/medical aromatherapy in London.

He was as good as his word, and on September 24, 1987, some thirty students gathered to pursue this exclusive training. On this occasion, Robert Tisserand came with his tape recorder and the interview I gave him then was subsequently published in Volume I, Issue No. I of a new periodical titled, the *International Journal of Aromatherapy*.

In order explain how the English (soft/Yin) aromatherapy is completely complementary to the French (hard/Yang) aromatherapy, I used an analogy in this interview that bears repeating today:

"If I can make a comparison with the world of plants, we in France are like the pollen; we have the yang aspect; we are very scientific. Here in Britain, you are like the ovula, the yin aspect. The conjunction of our scientific knowledge and your intuitive approach will make a beautiful fruit with many seeds inside." (IJA, February, 1988)

I have seen this vision of fertilization and mutual benefit realized over the past 11 years.

In 1988 Michael Scholes emigrated to the U.S. and settled in Los Angeles (where he still heads an aromatherapy training center with influence throughout the country). At his invitation and that of Marcel Lavabre, I continued teaching medical aromatherapy in annual visits to the U.S. from 1989 to 1991. During one of the first of these visits in 1989, I presented a day-long seminar to the American Aromatherapy Association (to which my wife and I have been named Honorary Life Members).[9] On this occasion I articulated the principles of what I call "Integrated Aromatic Medicine," (IAM) which has since spread throughout the world. One of the central concepts upon which IAM is based is my "Aromatic Triad."

The great modern figures in American aromatherapy attended one or more of these early seminars. One very significant meeting for us was with John Steele, well-known by all professionals and whose friendship is precious to us. Dr. Gary Young also attended these Los Angeles conferences. All the students who received French medical aromatherapy training at these conferences now hold key positions in the aromatherapy movement throughout the world.

In July 1990, after two years of intense work, the reference book, *L'aromathérapie exactement, [Exact Aromatherapy]* was published in France, issued as the result of work done in close cooperation with Pierre Franchomme over thirteen years.[10] In December of that same year, I returned again to Australia, where I taught in Sydney, Melbourne and Perth. A part of my heart will always be on this vast continent, but the mission on which I have embarked requires me to teach to the whole world.[11]

In 1991, most of my teaching was done in England at the request of various organizations. Rosalind Blackwell played an important role in bringing me into contact with medical herbalists. Robert Tisserand made it possible for me to connect with many people through three international conferences: Aroma '93, Aroma '95 and Aroma '97. Shirley and Len Price

have created a special course for aromatherapy, intended for health professionals, within which I have taught on the subject of "Intensive and Internal
Use of EO's."

Israel welcomed my teaching with great interest in April,1997, (spon-
sored by Mr Haim Schloss from Tel Aviv and Mrs. Charla Devereux from
Natural Oils Research Association, USA) and my seminars in Japan later
that same year (organized by Mr. Isao Tsunoda) were very successful and
confirmed the thirst for authentic information even in the Asiatic part of the
world. In a direct or indirect manner, the practice and doctrine of medical
aromatherapy, which started at the end of the 1970's, has now reached
most of the industrialized world.

This movement is irreversible. It will continue to unfold and change
medicine throughout the world. At this point, I am happy to have been
able to make an essential contribution to the worldwide expansion of
medical aromatherapy. But the task has only just begun. It is now necessary for all of us to organize together for the common good and future of
the planet. May I now share with you my thoughts on how we can do that?

Above all, keep a global vision, in time and in space. What do we really
want? This is the essential question, not only as it relates to our individual
success, but above all as it relates to the overall future of the world! We
are aware that essential oils constitute an extraordinary asset to help us on
both the personal and the world levels. Physically, emotionally, and spiritu-
ally, the impact of aromatic substances has turned out to be profound and
indispensable at a time of destructive chemical folly. Even the very large
laboratories know perfectly well that the natural health movement cannot
be considered a passing fancy, an ephemeral whim, or a transient fad.

The irresistible attraction toward essential oils and the extraordinary
development of aromatherapy worldwide constitutes a strong and beautiful expression of our innate instincts toward survival and conservation.

In a period of half a century, we have created an artificial, unnatural,
and now increasingly "virtual" world. Products and services that are
"chemically-engineered," "atomically-engineered," and "genetically-engi-
neered" involve real risks, some of which are known and recognized and
others which we are sadly continuing to discover. The destruction of our
environment is so advanced that I do not hesitate to compare our poor
Earth with the Titanic at the time of her collision: as water began to rush

through the break in the hull, the passengers continued their dancing and feasting on the bridge as if nothing had happened at all! We must stay acutely aware of one inescapable reality: we are all on the same boat. But contrary to the Titanic, there are no lifeboats with which some can escape disaster.[12]

Having taught thousands of students throughout the world, including directors of large organizations, I can see light at the end of this dark tunnel. I have a vision that together we can indeed create the radiant and prosperous future we all desire

The core of the message in integral aromatherapy is that we have a choice to respect, protect and love life. Millions of people in many countries are making that choice. This is what is behind the struggle currently being waged by thousands of responsible people in teaching, researching, producing, marketing and utilizing essential oils.

We can succeed together or perish together...the choice is ours and we must be fully aware of our responsibility in making this choice. Like the Titanic, our campaign for the recognition and success of medical aromatherapy, faces real dangers at this time. There are at least three categories of dangers, which individually are significant and in combination could be devastating. I call them...

the danger of "explosion,"

the danger of "dilution and dissolution," and

the danger of "implosion and dislocation."

The Danger of Explosion

An explosion results from an external attack: shells containing detonating charges are projected for the purpose of destroying a target.

Having been trained at a conventional medical school, I find myself in a very peculiar situation. On the one hand, I have great admiration and respect for the research and discoveries made in the various branches of medicine, surgery and intensive care. I know that any of us might some day see his life or that of his loved ones saved thanks to this scientific and technical medicine. It remains completely indispensable. At the same time, I know its limits and handicaps. The history of little Abby Bean given in her own words in the foreword of this book is one of the most striking examples of the failure of conventional medicine (and there are millions of similar cases of "artificial survival" under conventional medical care.)

The greatest present hinder to the spreading of medical aromatherapy is the total grip of the chemical-pharmaceutical industry on all teaching, research and medical practice. The moment corporate financial interests are allowed to determine the type and scope of treatment and/or medication, we begin to lose the spirit of true medicine. Let us not be naive about this situation. Largely because of financial interests, our present system will seek to preserve itself and assure its long-term survival. Natural solutions are usually viewed as competition.

Since essential oils are carriers of life force, builders of vigor and strength, and generators of calm and joy, they contribute powerfully to achieving and maintaining authentic and profound global health. It is easy to see that an impressive quantity of medications of all kinds could potentially be rendered useless or obsolete by these essential oils. This represents a profound threat to the chemical-pharmaceutical community, one that will be fought viciously in the name of self-preservation.

We should remember also that the most important thing, without a doubt, is that patients become more and more independent and responsible for regaining and maintaining their own health. I am reminded of the magnificent English word, which is difficult to translate precisely in most other languages, namely, "empowerment." In this context, it means giving to each person the power to manage their own health, harmony and well-being. It is implicit in the mission of integrated aromatherapy that we must educate individuals, families and groups in the regular use of essential oils.[13] The pharmaceutical industrialists are sufficiently intelligent to know that their real interest lies in supporting this great popular tendency to return to nature. But there will still be struggles to be waged and battles to be fought in order for this just and honest cause to triumph.

In order to defend itself, the aromatherapy movement should necessarily pass through a phase of internal restructuring, organization and regulation, in order to present to the general public a coherent image and to be able to speak forcefully, unitedly and clearly with the administrations and authorities of each country. This is a two-step transformation creating both internal support pillars (reorganization and regulation) and a protective external armor (consistent and professional dialogue with other organizations.) Currently, the United Kingdom gives the world a remarkable image of seriousness and responsibility. Another interesting example of internal restructuring and collaboration with administrative and governmental officials can be found in Australia and New Zealand.

Without the basic work–already on-going–of teaching, practicing and distributing essential oils, the aromatherapy movement would not now have the internal strength to withstand the inevitable attacks, and it would not now be capable of organizing for an adequate response. Remember, however, that in this struggle, our campaign is in no way directed against a system. It is, rather, a global concept and philosophy based on respect, synergy and symbiosis. We win as we integrate with existing systems.

The plant kingdom's best gift to the Biosphere and to Humanity is aromatic plants coupled with the human genius to create–through distillation–the birth of essential oils.

I know the day is coming when the medical use of therapeutic-grade essential oils will become a reality in hospital services; and the teaching of therapeutics using essential oils will be proposed and approved in numerous medical-pharmaceutical universities. I am aware of the great value of the preparatory work accomplished during all these years of patient research and passionate discoveries. For my part, I will continue to support the global and worldwide evolution of integral aromatherapy, provided I can work in the spirit of true medicine and with the attitude of harmony, peace and love that should uniquely characterize the aromatherapy movement. If we are to build the medicine of nature, our common beacon and our universal compass must be those values that are inherent in the natural Creation.

The Danger of Dilution and Dissolution

In an editorial in the *International Journal of Aromatherapy* (vol. 8, issue 4), Robert Tisserand wrote:

> "What is really sad is that so many people around the world have no idea what aromatherapy really is. They think aromatherapy is a hair spray which smells of hyacinth or a perfumed candle redolent of lily-of-the-valley."

If aromatherapy is confused with the artificial fragrances contained in mass-merchandised cosmetics, it will compromise the future of both the true science and the true art. If aromatherapy is reduced to these types of products, which typically come straight from petroleum chemistry, then there will be no hope for the millions of little Abbys throughout the world. No! Aromatherapy—particularly in its "hard" version with scientific and medical orientations—is, as its name implies and above all else, *a therapeutic form of medicine*. It does in fact involve caring for and saving lives.

In certain countries, the situation has already become so confused that we are going to see cigarette manufacturers, under the pretext of including menthol in their tobacco, claiming they are also doing aromatherapy! An incredible idea...but it must be recognized that the tobacco industry has no mercy or shame and is prepared to do anything to expand its lethal work, realizing billions of dollars in profits as it creates tens of millions of human cadavers. This is tantamount to genocide. The world record for the most odious industrial cynicism and outrage to the human family has to go to this industry, which unfortunately is an officially accepted one.

If aromatherapy is made popular by industrialists and corporate marketers, and is reduced to shampoos with artificial vanilla and soap bars that evoke a scent of jasmine, it will probably be necessary to create another name for true medical practice with essential oils in order to restore its true nature and make its mission respected.

To keep the public focused on real aromatherapy, it must be stated repeatedly that aromatherapy employs aromatic molecules in the form of genuine, therapeutic-grade essential oils to improve health. Artificial or adulterated scents have no place at all in this field! While smell alone is recognized as somewhat beneficial, it is only the very beginning of medical aromatic practice. When a suppository or a capsule containing essential oils is absorbed by the body, olfactory perceptions are practically non-existent, but therapeutic action is still very great.

The word "therapy," derived from the Greek and signifying "care," constitutes the key element in the word "aromatherapy." This care can be of a curative, preventative or developmental nature. In any case, there must exist a fundamental desire to provide aid and support to a person, an animal, a plant or even the soil, by making use of a natural substance extracted from an aromatic plant, mainly by means of steam distillation. The type of so-called aromatherapy we see in popular lines of cosmetics in retail shopping malls does not qualify for the name "aromatherapy." These products contain only minute amounts of essential oils, and then they are often adulterated, so there is little chance of realizing any therapeutic benefit from them. It is really little more than a recreational usage of scents and odors. We should call this "recreational fragrancing" and reserve the word "aromatherapy" for the real therapeutic use of authentic essential oils. If we do not succeed in re-establishing the correct sense for the word aromatherapy as conceived originally by R-M Gattefossé, then, as Robert Tisserand says in his conclusion, "...without powerful organizational representation, aromatherapy runs the risk of being consumed by its own success."

The Danger of Implosion and Disintegration

This is perhaps the most delicate and sensitive area to be addressed. But it is also the most critical one to enable us to resist external attacks (Danger of Explosion) and to resist corruption through artificial aromatherapy (Danger of Dilution and Dissolution). To better understand the problem of implosion, consider the process used to demolish obsolete or dilapidated buildings. Who hasn't seen the impressive images on television of imposing structures (especially in the U.S.) crumbling and collapsing on themselves!

To destroy a building by bombarding it from the outside would result in enormous damage all around the building and would entail great risk. The engineer's solution to this problem is implosion–placing relatively weak explosive charges at key structural points, so that the building is instantly deprived of its weight-bearing structure and literally falls in on itself.

When I consider the internal struggles currently taking place among aromatherapists worldwide, I cannot help but see the potential for implosion within our own ranks. These internal conflicts are undermining our essential support structures.

I want to pursue this analogy a little further, because it bears on our future just as critically as external attacks. Some of us have dedicated our lives and given all our love and the best of ourselves to the creation of legitimate aromatic medicine. It is deeply frustrating to someone like me to see "members of my own team" so to speak, arguing amongst themselves.

Imagine a structure resting on four pillars: its permanence depends on the strength and stability of each pillar. If just one of the pillars becomes weak, the whole building is in danger of falling. It is only as stable as its weakest pillar. Now, dear reader, I want you to imagine that this structure is a human being. To what would you compare the four pillars? Please close the book for a minute and ask yourself this question. Seriously, I would like you to put forth this intellectual effort and really ponder what are the four pillars that create stability for a human being? Please take a few minutes now, before reading any farther, and develop your answer to my question.

Now, let's consider your answers together. Do they focus on physical characteristics, such as the length of the intestine or the color of the skin or even the shape of the body and the appearance of the face? Have you confused the container with the contained? Or do you begin to see that there is something else beyond appearances and deeper than material structure?

As for me, if there is one thing I have learned beyond any question during my quarter of a century of medical practice, one fact about which my convictions are unwavering, it is this: *a human being is characterized above all else by the values of the spirit, and the pillars which create stability for a human being are spiritual pillars.*[14]

The four pillars of the human spirit, which provide almost invincible strength and power if they are solid, are the following:

1. The pillar of intellectual value = the TRUE
2. The pillar of emotional virtue and moral life = the GOOD
3. The pillar of artistic sensitivity = the BEAUTIFUL
4. The pillar of spiritual progression = the ULTIMATE ORIGIN and the living source of all values.

A stable aromatherapy—just like a stable human being—must rest on at least the first three pillars.

1. The intellectual approach to essential oils, through scientific knowledge, gives us a rational understanding of their action, which is necessary but not sufficient by itself.
2. The emotions and morality play a crucial role in directing the behavior and actions of all of us walking the aromatherapy path, whichever branch of it we have chosen; whether in cultivating the plants, distilling them, analyzing the essential oils, marketing them, creating synergies or families of products, teaching, or treating patients, the character of Goodness must be found at the center of all our thought and action.

3. The perception of artistic order and aesthetic experience give extra-ordinary personal satisfaction. This, in turn, reinforces the desire to better understand (creating synergy with the True), while support-ing good and just acts (synergy with the Good). With these three pillars, the edifice can stand solidly.

4. The fourth pillar, spiritual progression and order, although optional (it cannot be imposed on a person, but rather results from an intimate and profound choice within the consciousness) represents a type of supreme coronation linking us directly to the prime Source of all Values. This fourth pillar gives a much greater stabil-ity to the edifice and allows it to rise toward the highest peaks.

If the aromatherapy world chooses to unite its resources and build these invisible yet essential spiritual pillars, there is much to look forward to in the future. But if the petty fights for influence and personal interest, and the wars to win market share take the upper hand, despite the most elemen-tary morality, nothing and no one will be able to prevent the implosion. Should this occur, it will mean that we–who ought to know better–have failed to show the respect and harmony required by the world of aromatic plants. This is a crime of outright self-sabotage, a serious offense and the punishment we will receive–the loss of the opportunity to heal the world with these aro-matic medicines–will fit the seriousness of the crime. Justice will be done.

We are at a crucial turning point, but I have great hope for the future, and my hope does not rest on false illusions, but on real facts. This step of harmonization, of peace-making, must be placed at the top of our priorities. This message goes out to all my responsible friends. If I can be even a small catalyst in this reconstruction, particularly through the unique international position in which fate has placed me, it will bring me tremendous joy.[15]

Essential oils must lead us...to the essential

All involved in the great chain of love and devotion which begins with the cultivation and gathering of aromatic plants and ends with the act of applying the distilled essential oils for health treatment, must keep their spirits centered on this ultimate reality:

Aromatherapy carries a message of life and hope for tens of millions and perhaps for hundreds of millions of people.

I must confess, I am perplexed when I witness attitudes of hatred, misunderstanding and aggressiveness among a group of people who–because of the nature of their craft–should radiate harmony, inspire joy and exude peace. We are on earth to help each other and not to tear each other down, destroy each other, and ravage everything around us and finally ourselves! We must understand that even people toward whom we feel we have a right to hold resentment or anger have tried in their own way to contribute to the relief of suffering, in spite of any errors or mistakes they may have made.

A few weeks prior to this writing, the world witnessed an incredible reconciliatory event in Ireland. On May 10, 1998, after seventy years of merciless and horrifying fratricidal war, the people of Ireland performed, through a popular election, one of the most extraordinary acts of forgiveness and acceptance the world has ever seen. Each side accepted the other after so many horrors and crimes. Can aromatherapists rise to this same level? Can they meet with each other and through dialogue gain a better understanding and build unity through forgiveness? If Ireland can do it, surely aromatherapy can!

Whenever I get discouraged and doubt creeps in; when I sometimes wonder, "Am I right to dedicate so much effort and require so many sacrifices from my loved ones for the development of this ideal?" Then I start imagining how Abby, the little Australian girl, would have suffered through her medical and surgical Calvary without the help of essential oils. And in the end I must admit: "Yes, saving Abby–and creating the foundation for saving millions of other little Abbys–is well worth all the sacrifice!"[16]

To give myself the moral strength and mental clarity to finish the manuscript for this English edition in a very short time, I dialed Abby's telephone number just today and told her what joy I felt to be able to share her story with the great English-speaking public, beginning with North America. She was very touched to receive that unexpected call from 12,000 miles away. Her vigor and her strength are allowing her to pursue her studies brilliantly at the University of Adelaide, where she is majoring in speech therapy, a profession which will allow her in turn to make a great contribution to society. She knows how to use essential oils if a health problem arises and she told me how surprisingly fast aromatherapy and natural medicines are now developing in Australia. She is anxiously waiting for her copy of this book after its release this coming July. She understands how important this United States launch is for Rose-Marie and myself and told me that if the revolutionary wave of complete aromatherapy is starting in the U.S., it will reach Australia very quickly!

I quote now from her letter of May 16, 1996, in which she sent me her personal story which has become the foreword for this book,

"Writing it has made me realize just how much aromatherapy has changed my life for the better. Thank you, Dr. Pénoël...I am forever grateful."

And so, above all, I dedicate this English translation to all the little children like Abby throughout the whole world, as well as to their parents. I dedicate it to all my aromatherapist friends in all countries. And I likewise dedicate it to my colleagues in the medical and pharmaceutical fields and to all health professionals, nurses in particular, who are sincerely seeking the solutions that will give effective help and relief to the sick and educate them back to genuine health.

All of us together will build a better world.

Daniel Pénoël, MD

– I –

OSMOBIOSIS:
The Theoretical and Philosophical Foundation

INTRODUCTION

For the past 20 years, our lives have been intimately connected with essential oils. Working almost daily with these wondrous aromatic extracts has given us more experiences than we can count. They have taken us to the ends of the earth, including Australia, where we were able to demonstrate proof of their power.

Abby, a seven-year old girl from Auckland, New Zealand, had suffered from a serious respiratory infection since she was a baby. Within a month of her birth, on February 15, 1979, she began have problems. Prescriptions and antibiotics didn't seem to help. Could she be healed simply by leaving the humid climate of New Zealand and settling with her parents in the world's driest climate in Southern Australia? Could she escape her life of artificial survival, a life of permanent dependence on medication? Could she find instead a world of health and the joy of living? If positive answers to these questions were to be found, they would not be in a change of climate, but in a dream which first seemed impossible, a dream that brought my whole family to the land of eucalyptus and melaleucas.

Our migration is only one of our many aromatic experiences, but one that was lived with intensity and passion within our family unit and with the hundreds of patients we worked with in Australia. It is this experience that we wish to share with you through this first book. Let us discover together the world of Osmobiosis.

OBSERVE AND PONDER

Almost every theoretical model of psychological growth involves four stages. They have various names, but they are similar to the following:

1. Observe   2. Ponder   3. Decide   4. Act

When we first begin learning about something, we must process information, usually through the sense, in order to have an experience base upon which we can ponder or think about the meaning of those experiences.

It is common today to dispense with the spiritual and philosophical meanings behind the complex mysteries of essential oils. Too often the desire is only mechanical—"Just tell me which oil to use for arthritis..."—when there are deeper issues that ought to be explored. It is my great hope that when you are finished reading this book, you will feel a wonder and a reverence for these gifts of Nature. What makes them different is that they were not developed in a lab, they are not patented, no one own exclusive rights to them, and they are not new. Yet modern science is only just beginning to realize that they may be vital medicines for us in the 21st century. Whenever we approach something natural, we must, of necessity, be sensitive to the fact that it was created by an Intelligence far wiser than us. Reading this book should change your life. It surely will if you will try to get below the surface issues, go beyond the mere mechanical use of essential oils and get to the root of the matter. This will require all four learning stages: observation, pondering, decision, and action.

Part I of this book deals with issues that need to be observed and pondered before you can make intelligent decisions about aromatic care. By the time you finish Part I, you should have learned enough and meditated enough to be able to make life-changing decisions: decisions to expand your knowledge, skills, and wisdom about aromatic care; and decisions to accept the responsibilities inherent in using essential oils—not as mere chemical substances, but as Nature's complex gifts to make us more "alive." Having made these decisions, you will be prepared to act consistently and persistently in ways that will enhance your well-being, your harmony and your health.

Part II provides the information you need—the applications, techniques, recipes, etc.—to act correctly, confidently, and effectively in using essential oils to make your home and family healthier and happier.

ORIGIN OF OSMOBIOSIS

Osmobiosis is a way of observing, thinking, comprehending, deciding, and acting that enhances the life forces of the body. It is a mental "filter" that can alter our perceptions of all human existence and all phenomena in the living world. Osmobiosis is the term I use to describe the practice of natural care based on the use of aromatic plant substances, specifically, essential oils. But there is an important thought process behind such care that needs to be understood by both the care giver and the care receiver. Part I explains this thought process and philosophy.

Osmobiosis is a word I coined from combining two words, namely, "osmosis" and "symbiosis," and is the best way I could describe in one word the phenomenon of penetration and co-mingling of plant essences into the human essence.

My life has been dedicated to fighting pain and disease. In this fight, I have had thousands of experiences in "hand-to-hand" combat, as it were, to relieve human suffering, and they have laid the foundation for my philosophy of medicine and the way I approach any illness. It can be summed up in three simple words: life helps life!

The circumstances that gave birth to the concept of Osmobiosis began in April, 1977 when I opened my practice near Paris, following medical school. Seven years later, in April of 1984, we found ourselves in a difficult situation. I will not elaborate on the details, but suffice it to say that we had long wanted to spend time in an English-speaking country, and Australia was of particular interest to me because of its advanced research in essential oils, particularly eucalyptus and melaleuca. We had, in fact, applied for our visas to go there and I had left my Paris practice, but, unfortunately, our visas were denied. Then as if controlled by an unseen force, in a quick succession of events, political contacts were made in South Australia during a two-week trip, and we found a loophole in the immigration policy. Our visas to emigrate were approved in September, 1984, and we were given a short three months to move! There is an amazing story behind the story here, but that will have to wait for another book.

We felt directed–by friends and Providence–to go to Adelaide. In hindsight it seems this was not mere chance. One of our patients there, in April of 1986, was little Abby Bean, who wrote the foreword for this book. Her remarkable experience provides me with a foundation for illustrating the principles of Osmobiosis. So let me briefly tell you the story from my point of view.

For the first seven years of her frail life, Abby suffered chronic pulmonary, bronchial, and ear infections. Dozens of antibiotic prescriptions did not change her state of permanent infection. Worse, her physical and mental development had seriously suffered from this invisible, systematic attack on her body. Penicillin had brought on serious allergic reactions–her father himself had almost died following a violent reaction to a shot of penicillin–and the tetracyclines she had been taking had damaged her teeth, but left her infections alone!

She was like an old woman with arthritis, complaining of severe pain in her joints when the weather became humid. Her immune system, being disoriented by constants aggressions, finally turned itself on the tissues of the body. Her hearing had decreased, and she could not keep up with her classwork because she missed school regularly, every time her infections flared up. She was very thin and had no appetite for food or for life. She was at the mercy of serious relapses any time during the year. Abby was the only girl in her family, and her chronic illness created real desperation for her parents, Sue and Robert. After the apparent failure of allopathy, they consulted other kinds of doctors such as naturopaths, osteopaths and nutritionists, all without success. When an ENT specialist ordered an x-ray of the sinuses, it showed serious infection in the maxillary sinuses as well as the deep nasal cavities.

The specialist announced his grim decision to Abby's parents. He would proceed with yet another treatment of antibiotics for 15 days followed by another x-ray. If her condition had not improved by then, he would go forward with surgery, under general anesthesia, and break open the sinuses to release the puss and flush the nasal cavities. You can well imagine Abby's parents' reaction to this threat of further escalation in the "medical assault" against their darling little girl. It was the last straw for Robert. He announced to the specialist his firm intention to take a different course, to work with a new doctor and his wife who had recently arrived from Europe and been recommended by their osteopath. The specialist's response was sarcastic and threatening, "You do it at your own risk! And come back in two weeks with a new x-ray."

A challenge had been issued by the allopath. He had arbitrarily set a fifteen-day window for curing an infection that had festered under conventional medical care for seven years! During that seven years none of the medications prescribed for her had helped, except perhaps to make her condition more serious by shocking and weakening her immune system.

Thus we found ourselves facing a most complex situation and, given the specialist's disdain, our ability to resolve this situation would determine not only Abby's future well-being, but also the credibility accorded to aromatic medicine, being introduced for the first time in that part of the world.

Australia, like all countries under the Anglo-Saxon influence, knew aromatherapy as a practice for the relief of stress, by massaging the body with vegetable oils containing a few drops of essential oils. As pleasant and effective as this approach to relaxation and health maintenance might be, it was wholly inadequate in Abby's case. Her situation represented a true war zone. The therapy must be adapted to the severity of the illness, and even more important in this case, the diagnosis and treatment had to be correct in order to bring about a rapid recovery.

Conventional medicine could not properly comprehend Abby's problem. To say the cause of her pathetic condition was bacterial multiplication, to treat only the nasal cavities, and to fail to fully diagnose the cause of overproduction and accumulation of thick mucous can only lead to misdiagnosis and probable aggravation of the root problem. Abby symbolized the world of artificial survival in which thousands of tons of synthetic medicines (and millions of tons of other synthetic materials) are pawned on us annually, without ever giving us the power to create, promote, and maintain an exemplary and joyful state of health.

When the Bean family came to us, we set about immediately developing an aggressive plan of action. The steps we followed are part of the Osmobiosis philosophy. Our first task was to explain fully the reasons for the situation to Sue, Robert, and Abby. We were five partners with the three of them and my wife and I, joined in a common goal to mount a successful counter-offensive for Abby's health. This first step of explaining and clarifying was essential in order to determine whether the family had the necessary commitment to follow the difficult path back to health. When the "why" was understood, we started on the "how"–how to put in place a complete care program involving several complimentary steps or phases.

The first phase–nutritional correction–was the most important part of the treatment, because without it, the effect of the essential oils could be short-lived. Without nutritional correction, the action of the essential oils would quickly reach a plateau; improvement slows down and stops. Nutritional correction was necessary in order to give the essential oils every chance to have maximum possible effect.

A common mistake made the world over–especially with children–is to give them dairy products in abundance, usually in the name of supplying calcium. Fortunately this was not a problem for Abby, since her nutritionist had already advised Abby to abstain from all dairy products. Dairy products are in fact a major cause of overproduction of mucous, which in turn becomes a breeding ground for bacterial multiplication.

Part of nutritional correction is to objectively analyze present dietary habits. This sometimes requires great tact, particularly where children are involved. With wisdom, knowledge, and diplomacy, we proceeded to further analyze Abby's nutritional habits. This kind of work is well-suited to women, which is why my wife and I work together in a synergistic partnership. The Australian diet has some unique foods, unfamiliar to us in France. Among them are peanut butter and vegemite (a residue from beer-making). If these foods are only consumed occasionally, there is usually no problem, but when eaten every day, they overtax the liver and become difficult to metabolize. Their partially-metabolized residues find an exit out of the body through the respiratory mucous membranes, creating congestion.

These foods, along with several others, were easily observed as problem areas by my nutritionist wife. We reviewed several recommendations with Abby's parents and pointed out why it was important to consider not using certain foods anymore. Then we developed a complete nutritional program for Abby, including recipes that were not only healthy, but also tasty. We have learned that you cannot help a child with a weak appetite who has become very picky about her food if you do not have good-tasting recipes. We demonstrated and tasted the recipes with our patients in the clinic, so they would understand how to prepare them at home. Fortunately, Abby liked the new tastes of her nutritional program. She even agreed to drink carrot juice instead of orange juice (the "sacrosanct" morning beverage in Australia), which had been a source of de-mineralization in this gaunt little girl.

Strengthened by a basic knowledge of nutrition–an essential foundation for any serious and lasting program of therapy–we took Abby to the next phase: explaining the Intensive Aromatic Care (IAC) program. This phase, for her, included technical explanation and treatment with special equipment at the office plus a follow-up regiment to be conducted at home with the family. Every day after school, Abby came to the office for treatments of 1 to 2 hours. The treatments included aromatic aerosol therapy with sonic vibrations, magnotherapy, reflexology massage, manual and mechanical drainage, etc., which allowed us to work on the specific symptoms as well as her overall health. Robert, who accompanied his child, asked all the questions he wanted to about what the treatments were for and how to perform them. Working with Robert and Sue, we got Abby started on an intensive at-home agenda. This family enterprise consisted of three primary types of treatment: topical applications with essential oils, specially prepared drinks, and night inhalation of a directional mist. Abby and her parents worked well together to insure that these home treatments were performed properly and consistently.

This was the intensive program we followed for two weeks. After 15 days it was time to report back to the specialist. Although Abby's physical appearance was clearly improved, and she was obviously breathing better, we had no tangible proof of improvement in her sinuses. A great deal hung in the balance as Abby and her father went to the doctor's office on May 5, 1986. You can imagine their delight when the radiologist announced that all signs of infection–so prevalent on the x-ray two weeks earlier–had completely disappeared! For the first time in seven long years, Abby had shown significant improvement, and in only two week's time.

Robert and Abby were so happy they went immediately to the specialist to tell him the good news. His response, void of compassion for a child he had treated for years, shocked and deeply saddened Robert: "Cases of spontaneous healing are known to occur occasionally with children." When I heard this report, I felt like I was living in the Dark Ages, when the earth was flat and motionless, and the center of a universe was 6,000 years old, when people believed that blood did not circulate and there really was such a thing as spontaneous generation.

In short, surgery was avoided and aromatic medicine had proved itself on the Australian continent. For us and for Abby it was a tremendous victory. But the fight was not over. Abby had to continue her regular treatments and her nutritional program for many more weeks.

Three months after starting her treatment, we left Adelaide and moved to Melbourne at the end of July–the dead of winter in the Southern Hemisphere. At that point, Abby went through a short but quite severe period of tonsillitis, fever, and a cough. Looking at the case holistically, we did not conclude that a new "bug" had jumped into Abby's throat, but that her whole organism had gained enough strength, through the continued aromatherapeutic treatment, to expel toxins and waste matter that had accumulated from all her previous medications and infections. Every morning for four days an enormous quantity of thick brown mucus was found on Abby's pillow. To keep this acute elimination process under control (but not to counteract it), essential oils were used in the same intensive way as before, and after a battle of four days, her throat was completely cleansed, the fever had stopped, and Abby felt like a completely new person!

The official medical approach would have seen this four-day episode as an attack from an infectious disease. Seen through the light of holistic natural medicine, by contrast, it is understood as the body making its proper effort to continue and build on the work we had done for three months. Essential oils and a change in diet brought back vital strength to her body, which then–for the first time in a very long time–began working properly to heal itself.

As Abby's strength grew, she decided to proceed with a general cleansing through which all the toxins, accumulated during years of heavy medication, [of bacterial pollution and nutritional abuse], were evacuated. This kind of deep cleansing of the body systems created, at times, some severe but necessary reactions for Abby. An important part of aromatic medicine is understanding the meaning of these crises and learning to control them. Thanks to the strength of the essential oils and their ability to penetrate deep inside the body, we can recognize and respect these efforts made by the body to heal itself. Thousands of people every year can testify of the soundness and effectiveness of this type of natural medical approach.

After our departure from Australia, Abby continued aromatic treatments and followed a lighter, healthier diet. She is now completely symptom-free.

She is a beautiful young lady with a bright future. She is brilliant in her studies at the University of Adelaide, studying speech therapy. She likes sports, is a musician, and is very involved in preserving and protecting the environment. She has a great talent for writing, as you can tell from the foreword for this book. Having experienced firsthand a medical "resurrection" through aromatic medicine, we can expect to hear a lot more from her about it in the future.

When my wife and I think about little Abby and what she experienced in a climate much more agreeable than Paris, London or Detroit; surrounded by eucalyptus trees; in a country where life is much less stressful (even in school) than in Europe, it seems clear that even a pleasant culture and a healthy climate is not always sufficient to guarantee good health. On the other hand, aromatic medicine can allow one to achieve startling improvement, even when living conditions are not ideal. How do we explain this? Let's start by examining the principles of Osmobiosis.

THE PRINCIPLES OF OSMOBIOSIS

The Universe is structured upon certain great principles. It operates according to law, and we human beings must follow certain rules in order to combine with and be a part of the concert of the Universe. In our present society, many universal principles and their corresponding laws and rules are no longer taught in our schools and colleges. Today's students do not understand them because they are not aware of them. We might say they do not know that they do not know. Under these circumstances, is it any wonder that the world ecology is beginning to collapse under the weight of thousands of environmental pollutions that specialists can analyze, but cannot seem to control.

When we look upon the Universe as a whole, we can detect three successive levels of existence, namely Matter, Life, and Spirit. Each functions in its own sphere and mode of operation. But in each case we find Rhythm, Simplicity, and Harmony. What the human mind feels intuitively is confirmed entirely through the scientific approach.

The Beautiful, perceived through the senses, finds an echo in the True, discovered by the intellect, and the Good, conceived by our conscience.

The values, which after allowing for minor socio-cultural and ethnic varia-tion, can be seen as the foundation and the most precious heritage for humanity and the whole biosphere. These values are spiritual, and if they cannot be quoted on a stock exchange, we tend to forget them. We can see how far toward the destruction of the environment and our lack of knowledge and disregard for them has taken us.

The study of Life–the passage of Matter toward Spirit–is then, the most important course of study for widening our comprehension and enhancing the quality of our daily life.

From the standpoint of Energy, Life distinguishes itself from Matter by its aptitude to generate what scientists call "negative entropy." Entropy corresponds to the forces of death and decline, to the tendency toward decay, equalization, degradation, and descent toward the bottom. Iron rusts, batteries discharge, energy dissipates. It is a continuous "fall." In opposition to this tendency to decline, Life presents itself as islands of resistance to this process, the trend toward qualitative loss. If it is true, as Lavoisier explained, that "nothing gets lost; nothing gets created; every-thing transforms itself." The transformations that occur in entropy go toward a "minus," while the transformations that occur in Life move toward a "plus." Life shows itself as infinitely evolving and creative, a source of wonder and admiration constantly renewed. This "plus" makes existence better and greater, and should be the focus of a constant search for progress. The inventive genius of Life–its capacity for negative (or reverse) entropy–is profound even to the point that it has developed the means–through procreation and the genetic code–to reproduce and replenish itself.

As we examine the immense diversity of life forms, using one of the amazing gifts inherent in our own living process, namely thought, we can distinguish at least three categories of living things: those which produce, those which consume, and those which break things down and facilitate a recycling process. In this last process, death clearly nourishes life. But these cycles always begin with the capture and conversion by plants of a fraction of the solar energy which reaches planet Earth. Green plants are the sun-catchers of the living world.

The extraordinary phenomenon of photosynthesis converts electro-magnetic and light energy received on the surface of leaves and needles into biochemical energy. Through this process a great variety of complex molecular compounds are produced, including fats, proteins, cellulose, etc., which serve as the foundation of nourishment for other living things. Fairly recently in the earth's history (a few hundred million years ago compared to three and a half billion years since life first appeared), a very important phenomenon occurred: the evolution/creation of plant sexuality. This first appeared with the conifers and was followed by the evolution of our charming companions, the flowers, multicolored and perfumed, a source of constantly changing and renewing rapture. Nature continued to discover the value of the Aromatic Way in the plant kingdom, in the form of essential oils manufactured by various structures of many plants. Development occurred rapidly from that point on. A frenzy of spectacular creativity created unending variety. As of 1997, chemists had identified 70,000 different types of aromatic molecules, and new ones are being discovered every day! These molecules constitute the most concentrated and the most easily available form of combined Matter, Energy, and Information.

Herein lies the secret of the power of essential oils. It is this Aromatic Triad, carried by aromatic molecules (matter) imbued with energy potentials and information potentials unequaled in the living world, that penetrates into the core of the organism through Osmobiosis. We can better understand the workings of Osmobiosis through the following basic principles.

1. Life helps life.

The first principle of Osmobiosis is that through the application of essential oils, one can create the transfer of the Aromatic Triad–matter, energy, and information–into a human being. This transfer reverses the natural tendency toward entropy, i.e., it increases life's vital forces.

2. Osmobiosis is a habit, not an event.

The second principle is a logical corollary of the above transfer process. It is that aromatic matter is a life-sustaining and life-enhancing substance, which should be integrated into one's daily life, not reserved only for times when problems arise. Aromatic substances, including essential oils and floral waters, should occupy a regular and permanent role in home health care to enhance life, health, beauty, joy, vigor, and harmony. Like rays of sunshine lighting our path, aromatic substances enrich, expand, beautify, strengthen, and enlighten our lives here on Earth. Like jewels offered by the most highly evolved members of the plant kingdom, essential oils are pearls of life that contribute their infinite benefits to all those who understand the secrets of their power and who know how to use them with wisdom and consistency.

3. Aromatic matter must penetrate and integrate to provide its benefits.

The third principal inspiring Osmobiosis concerns the process of integrating the powers of aromatic substances into the core of the body. To provide maximum benefit, they should be applied through every logical interface (application method); having penetrated the body, aromatic molecules can integrate with the molecules of the body, becoming a functional part of the body. The very term "Osmobiosis" formed from the words "osmosis" and "symbiosis" expresses this penetration, co-mingling, and integration of both plant and human essences. The very nature of aromatic matter is providential: it is a fragrant liquid, acting immediately on both the conscious and unconscious systems of the brain. It easily penetrates the dermal layers, entering the blood and lymph systems to be transported throughout the body. Its therapeutic action is immediate, awe-inspiring–truly a small miracle. In this respect, the organ of the skin takes on great significance, requiring us to relearn the importance of tactile contact, touching, and massage.

4. The hand is the healer's instrument.

The fourth principle of Osmobiosis holds that the healer's hand is the tool which creates intimacy between the aromatic substance and the patient. The effectiveness of application with aromatic substances is largely dependent upon the skill in the healer's hands. The hand, when used properly with aromatic substances, can achieve a "non-bleeding surgery of the body and of the spirit." A re-learning of this art of the hand is a fundamental aspect of the Osmobiotic method, particularly because of the way it is used in the home, within the family.

5. Aromatic intervention starts intelligent healing.

This fifth principle concerns the attitude to adapt in the face of illness or injury, when one has a knowledge of aromatic medicine. The old adage of strict natural medicine to "let Nature take its course" is not part of the

Osmobiotic method. Besides being almost irrelevant in circumstances of accidental injury or trauma, this kind of thinking can be a philosophical obstruction to the relief and goodness Nature intended through providing aromatic medicines. In sum, this fifth principle can be explained as follows: Anyone who is in a position to stop or ease pain, reduce inflammation, resorb hematomas, prevent the spread of bacteria, promote tissue repair, accelerate a return to healthy function, or prevent unsightly scars–all through the use of aromatic substances produced by plants and extracted by man– should do so. Anyone who refuses or postpones such aid because of a doctrinal attitude is making a serious mistake. Even when the problem is not accidental, but the result of offenses (conscious) and errors (unconscious) against Life, immediate therapeutic intervention using aromatic materials is indispensable and appropriate.

Aromatic intervention provides reasonable relief while stimulating and supporting the Life Force within. It is grounded on, supported by, and prolonged through honest education of the patient.

6. Essential oils do not heal, but rather enhance the body's ability to heal itself.

This sixth principle concerns the proper visualization of how aromatic substances work. It is be implicit in all we have said thus far about essential oils, but to be perfectly clear, we make this explicit statement: essential oils are not the healing agents, but rather they are agents which promote the action of the body's own healing system. Remember that the body's healing system is much more than what we call the immune system. The immune system, although very important, is just one part of the body's total healing system, a vast ensemble of elements including the psyche, the nervous system, the endocrine glands, and other vital body systems. All can work together to heal and maintain health, particularly with the added support of essential oils. Through the Aromatic Triad (matter, energy, information) embodied in the oils, they are capable of providing help at many different levels, known and unknown, throughout the body's total healing system.

To better understand the therapist's role in administering essential oils, we can draw an analogy with the role of an orthopedic surgeon treating a fractured limb. His first task is to establish a complete diagnosis and then choose the best repair technique to align the bone and keep them in place.

The body then puts the healing system to work, starts the formation of new bone, and re-builds the bone, mending together the pieces. When the bone is sufficiently strong again, the patient can proceed to a phase of functional re-education or retraining and re-strengthening the muscles that move the bone. Finally, education and counsel may prove useful in helping to prevent future accidents.

The purpose, again, of the application of essential oils, is to mobilize all members of the body's total healing system. In this process the oils function like catalysts in a chemical combination, causing a reaction to start or accelerate faster than it would otherwise.

7. Essential oils, when used properly, create synergy at all levels.

The seventh principle of Osmobiosis admits to the reality of synergy surrounding the creation and use of essential oils. It exists at each level and in between levels. For example, the atoms in aromatic molecules work together in synergy; the aromatic molecules are found in essential oils in synergistic mixture; the complete oils are obtained through a synergistic relationship between Man and Nature with the matter designed and produced by the aromatic plant being extracted through the inventiveness of mankind. Human intervention becomes a synergistic influence also in the form of scientific and medical research done with essential oils as well as clinical therapy done with essential oils. These interventions bring about a synergistic marriage between the intelligence and intuition of Man and the creativity and wisdom of the aromatic plant world.

At another level, we can see synergy in the development of techniques for applying essential oils to increase their power to penetrate and to help the body's healing system. Integrating aromatic medicine into the core of mainstream health care will represent the synergistic optimum. In its broadest interpretation, the synergy envisioned in Osmobiosis occurs between Earth, Nature, and Man; hence its motto: Protect the Earth; Promote Life; Serve Man.

8. Essential oils are multi-dimensional in their characteristics, just as human beings are.

It is customary in medicine to speak of the "terrain" in which a problem or disease arises. This can apply to the operational health and/or weaknesses inherent in various body areas and systems. In a diabetic patient, the focus is on the pancreas and insulin production; in those addicted to alcohol or tobacco, the focus is brain chemistry and pre-dispositions; in the obese, the focus is on digestive processes and metabolism, etc. Each of us finds within ourselves varying terrains or body systems or functional realms—each of which is affected by heredity, nutrition, environment, and other factors. Some are strong, others have weaknesses; some are very responsive, others are sluggish. The great challenge is recognizing the intimate interrelationships that exist between these various realms. In standard medicine, efforts to determine these subtle and intimate inter-relationships are weak and sometimes non-existent. In natural medicine, on the other hand, we try to establish these relationships in addition to analyzing measurable symptoms.

In Aromatic Medicine, we take this to its logical extension, recognizing that there are many realms at work in the body, each one more or less suitable to receive a correcting or regulating influence from the essential oils. Further, we know that the oils are adaptogens in that they seem to understand—or the body understands—instinctively where their influence is needed and how it should be used. Thus it is important to understand that essential oils may provide therapy in unanticipated or unexpected ways, simply because they can have an influence in almost any system in the body. We will summarize here the realms in which essential oils can have an influence.

A. *The Congenital Realm.* Problems in this arena can arise from heredity or as a result of complications during pregnancy. Here, aromatic treatment can attempt to alleviate the consequences of problems irreparably written into the genetic code or of events from the time of conception until birth that have left a permanent developmental mark.

B. *The Organic Realm.* This refers to the actual organ systems of the body, including the liver, kidneys, lungs, spleen, cardiovascular system, digestive system, etc. On this level, aromatic molecules carry properties that promote improved functioning of the organs. Some of these properties have been studied pharmacologically and scientifically accepted. For example, eucalyptol is recognized as having a demonstratable beneficial action on the respiratory system. Consequently, a doctor, pharmacist, biologist, or any other scientific health professional who would presume to issue a disparaging opinion on the aromatherapeutic value of eucalyptol would find himself in contradiction with orthomolecular medicine. Such a rejection–in the light of scientific evidence–would be an obvious indication of ignorance, prejudice, or both. The basis of scientific investigation being objective intellectual curiosity, any refusal to study the science of essential oil therapy and any disparagement of its potential to provide valuable therapy is the equivalent of intellectual deceit. There is already too much evidence to the contrary.

There is the argument that double blind studies must be performed before valid conclusions can be reached. It is very difficult to apply double blind testing to Aromatic Medicine. Given the involvement of the senses of touch, smell, taste, and sight in the complete implementation of aromatic treatment, it would be a practical necessity for both the doctor and the patient to be in a coma in order to meet the theoretical requirements of double blind testing! By their very nature essential oils to not lend themselves to blind tests. On the other hand, we have frequently seen marked improvement in infants just weeks old after a few hours of intensive aromatic treatment. These infants, of course, were in no way subject to the power of suggestion–they could not even talk! They were in no way subject to the placebo effect because they had no understanding–even that they were being treated for a problem!

Millions of clinical cases treated by essential oils throughout the history of the world constitute "open tests" that a true scientific spirit cannot discount as mere anecdotal folk medicine. And hundreds of research studies are conducted each year in laboratories worldwide, which further verify the efficacy of essential oil treatments. Most doctors must at least admit their ignorance on this subject. Rather than criticize it, they should be more comfortable acknowledging that aromatic medicine is an entirely separate and extremely complex domain...one that will expand rapidly in a very few years.

C. The Bioelectronic Realm. Essential oils reveal an uncanny capacity to balance the pH, increase the electrical resistance, and reduce the oxidation within body fluids. In addition to this biochemical action of aromatic molecules, there is also their electromagnetic action, which can be very influential in creating an unfavorable environment toward pathogens.

We are today quite familiar with the harmful role of free radicals in the body. What is less well-known is that aromatic molecules have a power to somehow control and eliminate these free radicals, slowing down the aging process and even renewing the body. This action is readily noticed by those who make essential oil applications a daily practice.

D. The Microbial Realm. This refers to the flora and fauna co-existing with us in our bodies. We know now that within the digestive tract alone, we harbor more bacteria than there are cells in our body. This is something to think about when we know that among these "guests within" are our best allies and our worst enemies. Here we find an amazing property of essential oils in that–unlike antibiotics–they can be selective in their destruction of bacteria. They can preserve the good while eliminating the bad. Thus the corrective, purifying, and healing power of essential oils can be particularly profound in this realm.

I use the word "healing" without hesitation, because it has been proven through research that thymol, carvacrol, eugenol, and cinnamic aldehyde show antiseptic activity which is stronger than phenol. In its infinite wisdom, Nature has endowed each category of beings with its own defense system. By concentrating exclusively on antibiotics for half a century, mankind has totally focused on the lower plant world–that of mushrooms, mold, rot, or in other words, the family of decomposers and destroyers. Our mistake is not in the biological study of these microorganisms and their products, but in the systematic blind usage of them. The simplistic overuse of antibiotics constitutes a veritable abuse of power on the part of the entire medical profession. When a flu attack, which is purely viral, is bombarded with antibiotics, it becomes an unjustifiable waste of medicines. We know full well that antibiotics do not work on viruses. Antibiotics should be reserved for their specific targets. And even with bacterial infections, it is a sad illusion that antibiotics can cure all of them. Little Abby's sad story provides ample evidence of this fact.

But consider this simple and profound truth: the more highly-evolved families of the plant kingdom have also developed a means of protection from disease and infection. This means uses the form of aromatic molecules contained in their essential oils. It is now time for mankind to recognize and learn to use the higher level infection-fighting powers of essential oils. It is not only for their own benefit, but for the longer range benefit of the entire biosphere.

The microbial realm exerts a profound influence on the entire human body, including the psyche (numerous microbial toxins influence mood and morale). A large part of the universal action of essential oils lies in their ability to weaken the constant pathogenic aggression to which human beings are subject, while–at the same time–leaving friendly bacteria untouched. Antibiotics, by contrast, are not selective, destroying bacteria indiscriminately. We frequently see fungal infections start to proliferate, particularly candidiasis, after treatment with antibiotics (after all, antibiotics coming from fungus would favor other fungi). However, such manifestations never appear after treatment with essential oils. The entire human organism, physical and psychological, is strengthened and fortified, energized and revitalized, detoxified and purified from these amazing aromatic medicines.

E. *The Immunity Realm.* The importance of the immune system, and its profound effect on all other body systems is realized more every day. Here again, there are benefits from the universal action of essential oils. Aromatic treatments can be used to stimulate, regulate, or modulate immune system response, a function that is beginning to be recognized as medically invaluable. Once again, this is based on clinical research, not anecdotal case histories.

F. *The Structural Realm.* This realm relates to the bone, joint, and muscle systems of the body, in particular the spine, the axis extending from the skull to the tail bone. Often ignored by standard medicine, including rheumatologists, orthopedists, and occupational therapists, this realm nevertheless exerts a major influence on overall health as well as on the feeling of well-being. Although it would never presume to replace current corrective, energy, or structure techniques, aromatic medicine can play a support role that is extremely valuable. Because of the tactile and massage approach required for essential oils to penetrate the skin, the oils offer calming, pain relief, restitution, restoration, and relaxation in addition to stimulation or toning, depending on the oils used. In the context of natural home health care, this is where Osmobiosis finds its most common role. In the home is where the intimacy of touch can be enjoyed in the fullest sense of caring. Massage done regularly with essential oils at home on the body's structural systems brings benefits that have many positive repercussions for physical, nervous, and psychological health.

G. *The Glandular Realm.* This refers to the network of glands in the body which produce a vast and interrelated group of secretions to regulate most body functions and many psychological mechanisms. These secretions or hormones are–like essential oils–highly complex molecules which have a tremendous influence on the growth, healing, health, and regulation of body systems. Either by direct action or by more subtle biochemical processes (molecules which are precursors to hormone structures), essential oils can be used here also to stimulate, moderate, or regulate glandular performance. True, a destroyed gland or tumor require medical treatment or even surgery, but in less extreme cases, the influence of essential oils, when used regularly, will be clearly felt in a harmonious functioning of the endocrine concert.

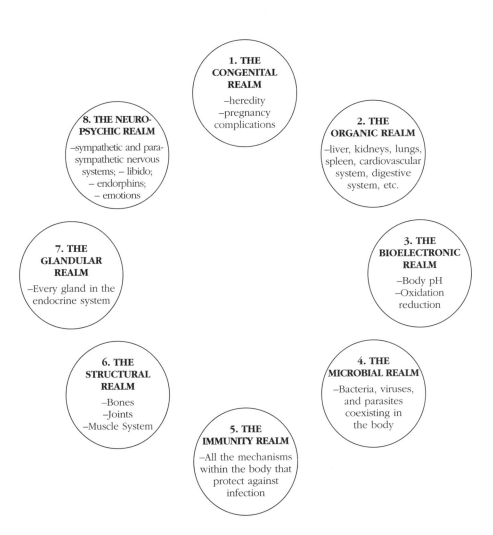

1. THE CONGENITAL REALM
–heredity
–pregnancy complications

2. THE ORGANIC REALM
–liver, kidneys, lungs, spleen, cardiovascular system, digestive system, etc.

3. THE BIOELECTRONIC REALM
–Body pH
–Oxidation reduction

4. THE MICROBIAL REALM
–Bacteria, viruses, and parasites coexisting in the body

5. THE IMMUNITY REALM
–All the mechanisms within the body that protect against infection

6. THE STRUCTURAL REALM
–Bones
–Joints
–Muscle System

7. THE GLANDULAR REALM
–Every gland in the endocrine system

8. THE NEURO-PSYCHIC REALM
–sympathetic and para-sympathetic nervous systems; – libido; – endorphins; – emotions

THE MULTI-DIMENSIONAL NATURE OF OSMOBIOSIS APPLICATION

H. The Neuro-Psychic Realm. This refers to all the functions related directly to and controlled by the human central computer, the brain. Pain response, controlling the sympathetic and parasympathetic nervous systems, production of endorphins, the functions of the subconscious and the memory, stimulation of the libido...there is no end to the list of nervous system functions that cannot be stimulated, moderated, or regulated by essential oils. This is one of the highest levels of response to aromatic molecules, and the fragrant nature of these molecules can sometimes have a profound and positive influence on the psyche.

This brief outline shows that Aromatic Medicine can be applied to every major body system. It is, in fact, a universal form of medicine, capable of helping in any biophysical realm. When all is said and done, it will become recognized as the medicine of harmonizing the systems, just as essential oils are in harmony with natural principles.

9. Essential oils do not change the soul.

This ninth principle takes a restrictive stance. Osmobiosis concentrates more particularly on the spiritual dimension of health (in contrast to the psychological dimension). The amazing influences of essential oils, particularly on the mind, have led some to believe that they had mystical powers and that those who used them were in some way "spiritual masters." Both of these notions are seductive traps. They have no part in Osmobiosis.

If all you had to do to become Saint Teresa of Avila or to be transformed into St. Francis of Assisi was to obtain the queen of essential oils–that extracted from rose petals–then heaven could be bought with money. Thank God that is not the case. Spiritual development knows no shortcuts. It results from a conscious and voluntary effort on the part of each individual. There are gymnastics for the soul just as there are for the body.

Muscle stimulation by electrical impulses, even if you use the most expensive and the most perfect device available, cannot compare to the effects of a real physical workout, with its beneficial results for the heart, lungs, brain and–perhaps most important–the will. It is the same with spiritual development. Essential oils bring untold benefits of all types, but one must avoid attributing any pseudo-mystical powers, inspiration, or extra-terrestrial connection to aromatic medicine. This is a scientific endeavor, based on research, to find truth. It must not be relegated to self-proclaimed mystics.

Humility, patience, open dialogue and respect for different approaches and different practices–these are the qualities that must characterize the researcher in Aromatic Medicine.

10. Make the Earth our garden.

This tenth principle expands all the fundamental concepts of Osmobiosis into the entire biosphere. It creates a vision for what can happen as more and more families throughout the world–both in developed and developing nations–learn about and begin to practice the Osmobiotic method. It is easy for us to see that a time is coming soon, when aromatic medicine will become so popular that current sources of essential oils will be wholly inadequate. If we do not begin, properly cultivating new resources for essential oils now, we will be unable to obtain high quality, unadulterated essential oils at a time when we most need them.

AIDS, Chronic Fatigue Syndrome, new aggressive strains of STDs, malaria, and cholera, are all clear danger signals. To get on the right track, we must depend more and more on research independent of conventional medicine and conventional medicine's financial fortunes. Our present medicine system is guilty of serious mistakes and gross misconduct in the way it deals with the biosphere as a whole. If we continue to research and treat only symptoms instead of causes; if we work to bring about temporary relief instead of permanent cure; if we forget to look at the causes of the causes, then there is a real possibility that these new trends in uncontrollable disease will expand. What we see now as a concern below the surface will erupt in a worldwide devastating fury.

The philosophy behind Osmobiosis requires a new perspective of the Earth, Time, and Man. Consider for example, the acreage being devoted to crops of death, such as tobacco, alkaloid plants used abusively (coffee, tea, cacao), crops for "illicit" drugs (marijuana, heroin, etc), and crops grown to create refined sugar, another devastating "drug." The total of all this acreage is truly immense. Think of the impact that would be created if these areas of the earth's surface were partially and progressively converted to grow and produce aromatic plants from which essential oils could be produced! The Aromatic Biomass, or all of the aromatic molecules produced annually by the aromatic biosphere (all plants that produce essential oils), constitutes a vital resource whose time has come for evaluation and review by mankind.

There are major implications for the quality of life on earth inherent in this evaluation. We can make the earth a vast garden of health, of phyto-medicines (plant medicines) that will expand our personal health and the health of the whole biosphere. This paradigm shift begins with individual and family awareness. Hence the importance of learning natural home health care with essential oils.

SUMMARY OF THE TEN PRINCIPLES OF OSMOBIOSIS

1. Life helps life. The life force–Matter, Energy and Information–carried in the aromatic-substance is transferred and integrated into the human body, reversing natural entropy.

2. Osmobiosis is a habit, not an event. Essential oils are life-sustaining substances which should be integrated into one's daily life.

3. Essential oils must penetrate to provide benefit. Every logical interface can and should be used to help the aromatic molecules penetrate and integrate with the human body. Osmosis + Symbiosis = OSMOBIOSIS.

4. The hand is the aromatic healer's instrument. The aromatic healer's hand is the tool which creates intimacy between the essential oil and the patient.

5. Aromatic intervention starts intelligent healing. It is appropriate anytime benefit can be delivered; it soothes intelligently; it addresses causes rather than symptoms; it stimulates and supports the Life Force, and it is supported by careful education of the patient.

6. Essential oils do not heal, but enhance the body's ability to heal itself. Essential oils are not the healing agents, but rather they are agents which stimulate the action of every facet of the body's total healing system, including–but not limited to–the immune system.

7. Essential oils embody synergy at all levels. The Osmobiotic perspective is that all things can be seen as working together for the common good. Our motto expresses this at its highest level: Protect the Earth. Help Life. Serve Man.

8. Essential oils are multi-dimensional. The fundamental multidimensional nature of essential oils responds and adapts itself to the multidimensional nature of human beings.

9. Essential oils do not change the soul. Aromatic care is not "mystical" and those who administer it are not "spiritual masters." It is a healing endeavor–both scientific and artistic–that can be learned by all.

10. The earth can be an aromatic garden. The philosophy behind Osmobiosis requires a new, positive perspective of the Earth, Time, and Man. When we use the biosphere to create an aromatic resource rather than to produce "crops of death" to make money, the earth indeed will become an aromatic garden.

OSMOBIOSIS APPLICATION LEVELS

Osmobiosis has developed from a long list of exciting concepts. It goes beyond merely applying natural medicines and embodies a total philosophy and methodology of care based on moral values. It can be used in a full variety of situations, from mild to severe. Its beauty is that, when necessary, it can be particularly aggressive in fighting serious disease and infection. It is a broad methodology that can be appropriate even in dangerous situations. We have developed techniques to push the cleansing and revitalizing influences of essential oils to extreme levels in critical cases. Consider the aggressive care given to Abby: hundreds of these types of situations, pathological and accidental, have arisen in which the efficacy of essential oil therapy has been proven. In the context of natural home health care, aromatic medicine can be used in simple, daily ways to create general well-being, health, and harmony, but should the need arise, intensive aromatic applications can also be used in emergencies.

Other fundamentals of aromatic care include the following:

1. In order to do their healing work, essential oils must penetrate to the very core of the body.

2. When we examine how the body works, we see that the internal parts of the human body come in contact with the outside environment through three primary interfaces:

the skin

the respiratory membranes, and

the digestive membranes.

Each of these interfaces or contact points has its own ability to receive and transform the aromatic molecules in essential oils, and diffuse them toward the interior of the body. For most of the applications involved in natural home health care, the primary interface or penetration route is the skin.

3. One cannot indiscriminantly use any essential oil on any interface in any concentration with any carrier. Each essential oil has unique characteristics that determine how it will respond with each of the different interfaces.

4. Because essential oils are life substances with broad potential for positive action (and not prescription drugs with narrow and specific activity), they can be incorporated into daily life with ease, simplicity, and relative safety.

We specify three levels of intensity in our aromatic practice:
1. Regular Aromatic Care or Aromatic Discipline (RAC)
2. Emergency Aromatic Care (EAC)
3. Intensive Aromatic Care (IAC)

The first two of these three levels can be learned by anyone and should be part of your natural home health care. Level 1 involves simple daily procedures to enhance health and well-being. Level 2 is needed for emergencies that occur every day at home, but are not serious enough to involve a hospital. Level 3 is usually administered by a trained health professional. The intensity of this care level requires intimate knowledge of essential oils and their interface relationships. This is the type of care that was administered to Abby.

A knowledge of RAC and EAC can often bring immediate relief and prevent complications which might otherwise develop. We should also point out that when essential oils are used in daily hygiene, it is far more likely they will also be used in urgent situations.

In summary then, Emergency Aromatic Care builds on the foundation of Regular Aromatic Care. The daily impact of RAC provides regular harmonizing, fortifying, and rejuvenating, while Emergency Aromatic Care (and Intensive Aromatic Care) are added when intervention is needed for sudden and/or serious disease and injury. These more intensive care levels may last for hours, days, or weeks as the situation may require. And when complete, their beneficial effects are maintained as the Regular Aromatic Care regimen resumes.

A great deal of practical information about these three modalities, including application instructions with specific essential oils for specific problems is included in Part II of this book. Before starting that area, however, we would like to elaborate further on each of these modalities to create a clear understanding of the differences in style and philosophy that pertain to each one.

Regular Aromatic Care (RAC)

Also referred to as Aromatic Discipline, RAC encompasses the daily use of essential oils for general prevention, vitalization, well-being, and harmony. It finds its perfect setting in the home, therefore becoming the foundation for natural home health care. It is supplemented by more urgent and intensive care when sickness or accidents require.

A proper RAC regimen involves at least two daily "episodes" or treatments with the oils: morning stimulation and evening relaxation. The details of these treatments are explained in Part II. In this context, essential oils can be used singly, but for superior efficacy, experience has shown that essential oil blends, when properly formulated, create indispensable synergy. The key advantage of blends lies in their harmonic creativity and subtle compensations, which prevent the human body from becoming dependent on them. Using the essential oil of lavender or one of its hybrids for relaxation can be pleasant for several days, but when used by itself daily over a long course of time, the result can be physical laxness and a relative loss of the desired effects. In contrast, by using blends that have been carefully researched and tested, and which combine a rich variety of complementary aromatic molecules, tendencies toward dependence are avoided. The full effects of the essential oils continue even after a period of lengthy use.

Another consideration about blends: within the context of RAC, one can create subtle "variations on a theme" by making modest variations in the oils used, the dilution level, and in the proportions of the constituents. In this experimentation, Man, following the example of Nature, becomes an aromatic co-creator, combining his intelligence and intuition to respond to specific needs.

The most critical requirement–and the most difficult re-learning–which must take place for RAC is *the discipline to use the oils regularly each day*. This is a habit that can be difficult to establish, so I offer some important observations here on page 69 under the heading "Decide."

Emergency Aromatic Care (EAC)

This is the 'first aid' of aromatic care. Despite our expanding civilization and amazing technology, life in our modern world still brings a great many circumstances where we can experience physical and psychological trauma. More than ever, we need to recognize the increasing frequency of mental and nervous "attacks" and difficulties. The key to EAC, of course, is preparation. In any emergency or first aid situation, the remedy must be immediately available. So it is with EAC. A basic collection of aromatics, which can be used in a wide variety of first aid cases, should be assembled. This is a basic starting step in the practice of Osmobiosis.

This aromatic "first aid kit" is important in more than one way. It enables rapid response to promote immediate healing. But immediate response also frequently brings immediate relief, which in turn brings immediate confidence in the efficacy of the treatment!

This effect is best learned and experienced through a typical emergency example: a blow to a bone surface, especially in the less fleshy regions–the iliac wings (edge of the pelvis), the elbows, or shins. A sharp impact on these areas typically results in considerable pain. A dramatic reduction in the pain is immediately seen after an initial surface application of the right essential oils. Later supplementary applications may be helpful, but typically the initial relief is long-lasting and completely sufficient for minor accidents. In addition to this immediate analgesic effect, a similarly remarkable action can be seen in the rapid recovery of any injured tissue. Immediate application for pain also helps prevents inflammation, which could be a starting point for more serious complications. Anyone who has had this experience has been completely convinced of the power of essential oils for first aid treatment.

Emergency Aromatic Care should be included in all first aid training. I am confident that one day soon, aromatic first aid will indeed be a basic part of first aid instruction, not only for medical and paramedical personnel, but also for children and families.

We have "cheated" the laws of life for decades, consciously or unconsciously, as victims of a short-sighted system which creates "remedies" that do nothing more than suppress the physical intelligence (symptoms). When you think about how long we have been doing this–looking for the quick fix, treating the symptom instead of the cause, and ignoring the inherent healing system of the body–it is no wonder that degenerative diseases are running rampant. Their absence would be a greater surprise than their presence.

Aromatic Care in any of its levels sustains the laws of life, rather than cheats them. It borrows from some of the highest powers of the plant kingdom and makes them available to human and animal life. Once we have obtained the education to administer the blessings of these wonderful aromatic molecules, it is not an obligation, but rather a privilege to be able to use them. In Emergency Aromatic Care, intervention with essential oils is like a peak, a brief and intense point on the graph of aromatic time. If the intervention needs to be prolonged for several hours, days, or weeks, it then enters the realm of Intensive Aromatic Care.

Intensive Aromatic Care (IAC)

When it is clear there is a need for repeated strong aromatic applications over time, regardless of the interfaces involved, IAC procedures are indicated. This need arises typically in two types of situations:

A. A sudden and severe acute state, usually a bacterial or viral infection, requiring a quick counter-attack. Intensive aromatic care will help set in motion all the healing resources of the body. Particularly important in these cases are the synergies found with essential oil blends.

B. A long-standing chronic problem, for which the caregiver has decided to create an aromatic shock designed to shake up the 'torpor of life force' and break a vicious cycle. IAC is the springboard which can create a temporary phase of organizing chaos, followed by the re-establishment of the body's own life force.

Abby's case illustrates both situations. When we first began treatments in April, 1986, hers was a chronic case requiring a breaking of cycles and a new re-vitalization of the body's forces. Three months later, in July, at the time of her last eliminative crisis, her situation was an acute attack. In both instances—due largely to her family's resolute determination, the core of all healing—the treatments were extremely successful...as they have been in thousands of other cases.

Significant quantities of essential oils are required in IAC, in order to create a literal whirlpool of aromatic matter, energy, and information, penetrating the body at regular intervals over an extended period of time. This subjects the enemy (disease or injury) to an aromatic fire which is regularly re-fueled until the enemy is completely destroyed, with no chance of escaping and reappearing later in another part of the body.

For serious pathological situations, IAC requires the direction of a therapist trained in the tactics and strategies of aromatic medicine. Ideally, difficult cases should be treated in Aromatic Care Centers.

DECIDE

Both in my clinical practice and in my teaching, I see over and over again that most people have great difficulty modifying their daily habits and persevering in such changes until new habits are formed. I believe this grows out of a mistaken belief that adequate results can be obtained without making a permanent change. Let me share my view on the problem.

If you are experiencing health problems; if you have fallen ill and remain so; or if the same problems recur frequently, it means something is not right. Before blaming the outside world–which generally will not change–it is wiser to make an about-face, look at the inside world, and analyze the elements in your own life that are susceptible to change, looking for incorrect behaviors and attitudes that need correcting.

If we continue to think, speak, and act as we have always done, we shall continue to reap the same things we have always sown. It is critical that we face the music on this issue, acknowledging our faults and weaknesses in order to give us a deeper motivation for change, a motivation that will be great enough to insure success in altering our basic life habits.

The tremendous advantage of essential oils lies in their capacity to open our consciousness and influence positively our efforts to change and improve old life patterns. This can apply in our attitudes towards others as well as in our daily habits. In Part II of this book, you will receive a sure and firm guiding hand to help solidify your desires for change. You will find a step-by-step approach that will help you integrate aromatic thinking into your whole life. Through it, you will achieve your aspirations to be better and live better. I know you will reap the most beautiful and delightful fruits you can imagine from your attentive, regular, and persistent care of the Tree of Life and its nourishing soil.

Footnotes

1. I have now worked for two years with the EO extracted from **pelargonium tomentosum** (which I have given a common name of 'mentholated geranium,' and this new EO was presented in my book, Urgences et Soins Intensifs, to be later translated and published in English.

2. Australia is one of the strictest countries in the world for the granting of permanent immigrant visas. It truly required enormous tenacity and a large portion of the "Australian dream", which still exists in the collective subconscious of many French people, to succeed in obtaining a visa for the entire family after three years of struggle. The true "novel" of this Australian adventure will be published later.

3. Don Gary Young presented two topics on the occasion of this symposium: the medical application and home uses of essential oils; and the practice of organic farming; and new techniques for steam distillation.His high-quality presentation was greatly appreciated by all the participants

   The presentation of the clinical case of the total healing of a malignant tumor in the neck was particularly impressive and touching. The presentation of the work accomplished in agriculture, involving the use of aromatic plant extracts for care lavished on the soil and on plants strengthened my conviction of the concept of total biospheric aromatherapy: providing the same loving care for the nourishing earth, plants, animals, and human beings. The technical perfection brought to the distillation for obtaining high quality therapeutic essential oils clearly takes into consideration this intimate relationship between the creative genius of the aromatic plant and the inventive genius of the human being. Thank you and bravo for this wonderful contribution!

4. It is simply a statistical finding and it is certain that these situations are bound to evolve in the near future, on one hand with the European Union and on the other hand with "globalization". This geographic differentiation has been globally acceptable up to the present.

5. One of the most beautiful symbols of this "caring" attitude is without doubt the life and work of the nurse Florence Nightingale. A reference to this limitless devotion is rightly given in the beautiful book written by Jane Buckle: "Clinical Aromatherapy in Nursing", which I had the opportunity to read before its submission to the printer, on the occasion of our meeting at the Shirley Price College of Aromatherapy in September 1997 (Arnold publisher, 1997).

6. It should be noted that Germany represents in itself the only large European market for medicinal plants and where natural medicine is officially practiced by "Heilpraktiker" (non-medical practitioners). Biological agriculture is practiced at an intense level, and most baby foods are prepared from biological products. In other respects, the major aromatherapy laboratories in Germany are extremely strict regarding the quality of essential oils. It is sometimes a pity, in my opinion, to see essential oils of such biological and therapeutic value simply go up in smoke in "aroma burners".

7. Robert Tisserand has played a large role in making the work of Dr. Jean Valnet known to the Anglo-Saxon world, and from there to the rest of the globe. It was he as well who took it upon himself to translate into English the book written by René-Maurice Guttefossé. He was therefore instrumental in the origin of a very important "bridge" between France and the English-speaking world, and in parallel and complimentary fashion, in the construction of the "tunnel of scientific aromatherapy" which has allowed the English-speaking world to become familiar with a form of aromatherapy which is far more precise in its molecular understanding and much more demanding in botanical knowledge and in the quality of essential oils.

Dr. Jean Valnet (born 26 July 1920 and died 29 May 1995) will remain as a great figure in medical aromatherapy integrated in a large practice of natural medicine. He always realized the importance of the quality of essential oils to guarantee the best results, even if, during the time of his own activity, the market did not provide this necessary quality. The current evolution of the production of high quality has enabled the laboratory which he created to be in a position to propose a range of essential oils for family use offering guaranteed biological quality. What a wonderful validation after so many years of struggle!

8. Henri Viaud, a professor of mathematics, turned distiller of aromatic plants, has played a great role in the training of numerous pioneers renowned in aromatherapy. He has rightly been chosen as honorary president of the First International Symposium of Integrated Aromatic Medicine at Grasse.

9. On the occasion of a trip by car between Los Angeles and San Francisco, Michael Scholes had us meet in San Jose, the world software capital, with a group of people who had gathered around a woman who had gifts of perception as a medium, or as is said in the US, a "channeling person."

This woman, who had not heard anything in particular about aromatherapy (this happened in 1990), suddenly "received" a message concerning me, which she expressed thus: "With you, a new aromatic language is coming to America"! The appropriateness and truth of the message can be understood better by considering the fact that the conceptual approach, which will be developed progressively in the works in the collection "Integrated Aromatic Medicine," implies especially a planetary, global, and temporal-spatial vision that gives a particularly original dimension to the system and the method.

10. F. Franchomme and Dr. D. Pénoël: *L'aromathérapie exactement* [Exact Aromatherapy] (Editions Jollois). Not translated into English at present.

11. On September 27, 1986, a critical event would occur in Melbourne: the meeting with Leslie Kenton, an author who is well known, especially for her books on natural nutrition.

Her message regarding me was very clear: Dr. Pénoël, your mission for the world is too important for you to stay in Australia. You must be back in Europe!" And she really played a very large role in enabling me to return to France in February 1987. This meeting was not the result of chance, but of the pursuit of accomplishing my "life mission."

12. Speaking of icebergs, it must be recalled that what we perceive as the current state of ruin and devastation of the planet only constitutes a very small fraction of the reality, which is more somber and more threatening that we imagine!

13. During our travels, we have trained clients several times. When we have had to leave our patients, they evidently regret our departure, but they have learned how to make do alone, with essential oils and natural medicine, for most current problems, and this is for us the best criterion to be met according to our ethics, which are based on the transmission of knowledge and the learning of know-how.

14. This conviction is shared by numerous researchers throughout the world. Norman Cousins, in the United States, has played an important role in the heightened awareness and the living demonstration, typically American, of the decisive influence of the spirit. The best-seller *Anatomy of an Illness* is surely well known among English-speaking readers. The audio program K7, entitled "Head First" (the Biology of Hope), published by Nightingale [Conant] Audio (R) is a remarkable complement to the book. Psycho-neuro-immunology is playing a bigger role in modern medicine, and all aromatherapists know by experience that a large part of the action of essential oils also passes through this channel.

15. At the time of the international event constituted as AROMA 97, organized by Robert Tisserand, a general assembly was spontaneously organized in which all the representatives were able to express their wishes to harmonize the aromatherapy movement on a global scale.

This experience was felt with an intense emotion and a profound joy by all participants. The fact of having been able to organize the first Integrated Aromatic Medicine Symposium in the city of Grasse also represents a big step and a very encouraging sign for the future of and the integration of France into the international movement.

16. My wife, who has had many uncommon adventures because of my passion with aromatherapy, unfortunately sometimes has had sad experiences that led her to say, "It's no longer aromatherapy; it has become aromathera-pew!" (In French, "Aromathérapue," where "pu" means "stink," which is the exact opposite!).

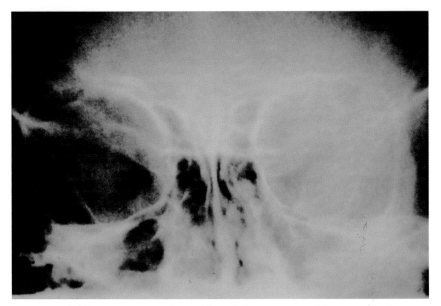

1. X-ray of Abby's sinuses on April 17, 1986. Radiologist comment: "There is mucosal thickening and air fluid level in the right maxillary antrum. There is quite extensive mucosal thickening about the left antral walls. The ethmoid and rudimentary frontal sinuses appear reasonably clear and the sphenoid sinus that has developed is also well aerated. There is a large adenoid soft tissue mass which appears to obstruct the naso-pharyngeal airway on the lateral view. There appears to be some leftward bony nasal septum deviation and the nasal airways appear a little obstructed by prominent turbinates."

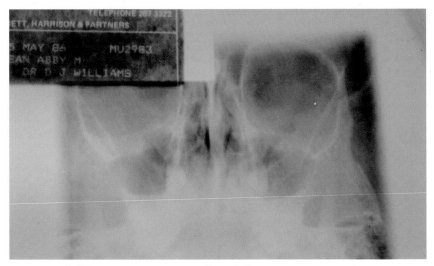

2. X-ray of Abby's sinuses on May 5, 1986. Radiologist comment: "A single Water's view shows the maxillary antra to be clear which indicates marked improvement particularly to the left side."

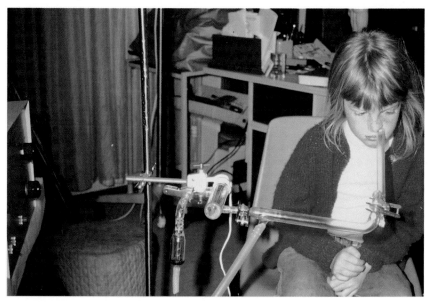

3. Abby receives her daily aerosol session in Dr. Pénoël's office in Adelaide.

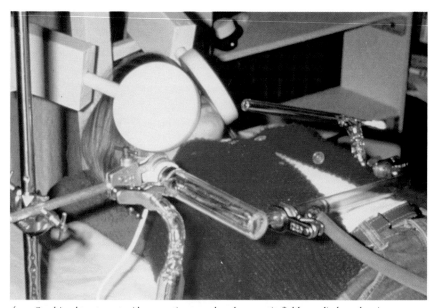

4. Combined treatment with aromatic aerosol and magnetic fields applied on the sinus areas.

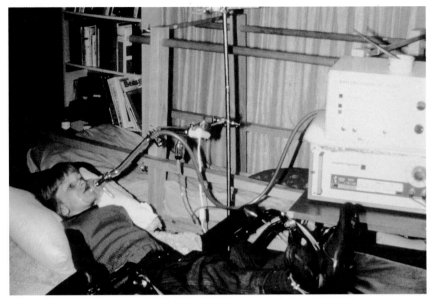

5. Aromatic aerosol session using a mask on the face. Abby is already looking better.

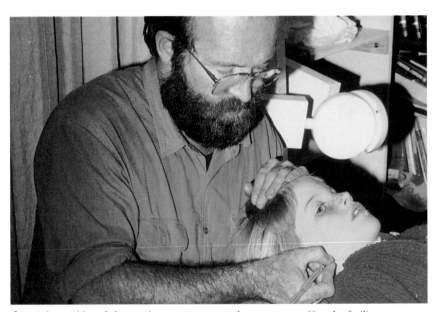

6. Robert, Abby's father, took an active part in the treatments. Here he facilitates drainage along the face using surface suction.

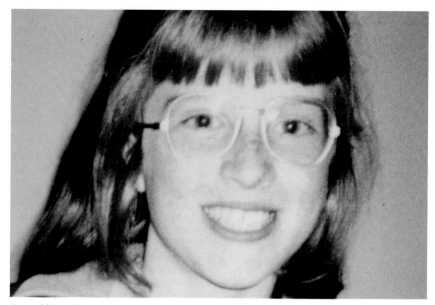

7. Abby at the age of 13: a healthy and happy young lady. Since her treatment, she has not taken any further antibiotics to this day.

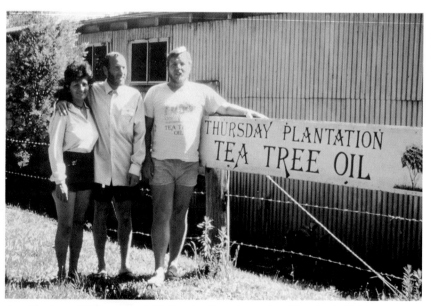

8. Christmas, 1986, spent with Christopher Dean in northern New South Wales, Australia. Dean has played a major role in the agricultural development of the tea tree industry in Australia.

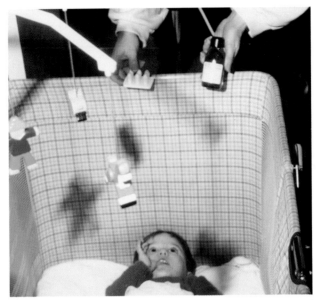

21. The Osmobiosol® has been set up above the bed of this young child, so she can breath a fine aromatic mist during the entire night. Her parents were so pleased with the results that they purchased the system for permanent use in the home. Only premium quality essential oils should be diffused in this manner.

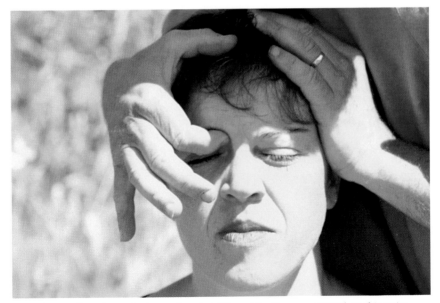

22. The "ouch" point at the internal angle of the orbit. Pressure exerted on this point, moving from the outer edge of the eye to the inner edge (near the nose) triggers a pain in most westernized people. Once the cleansing program has been seriously implemented, the pain goes away.

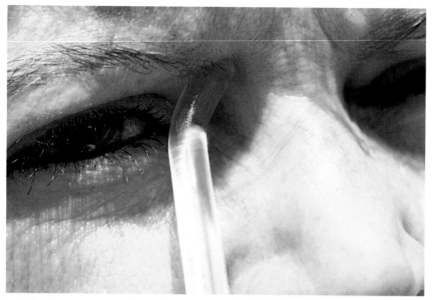

23. Exerting pressure on the "ouch" point, using a curved glass rod.

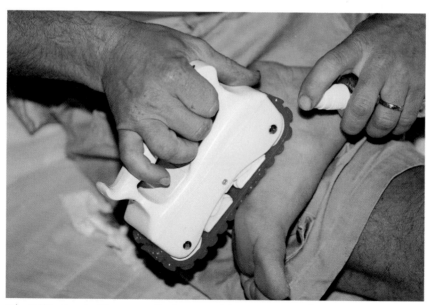

24. Self treatment with rosemary floral water and Supra Spirex on reflex points of the left foot.

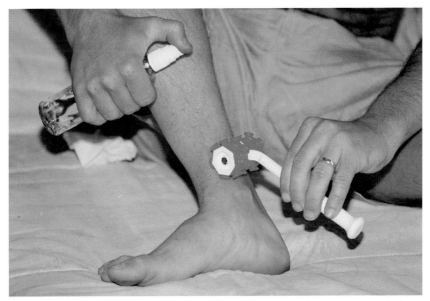

25. Dr. Pénoël applies the Facial Spirex and floral water to a tender area (where it had received a sharp blow) to unblock "microcrystals" that have formed in the tissue. Three sessions of 20 minutes will completely relieve the situation.

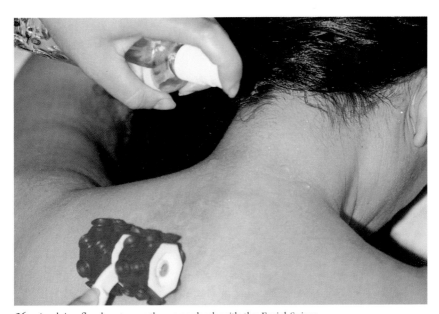

26. Applying floral water on the upper back with the Facial Spirex.

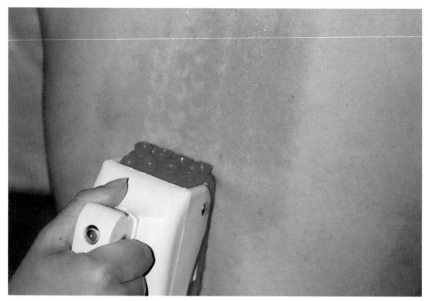

27. Back massage using the Supra Spirex and floral water. The marks left by the suction cups are clearly visible. This treatment is very relaxing.

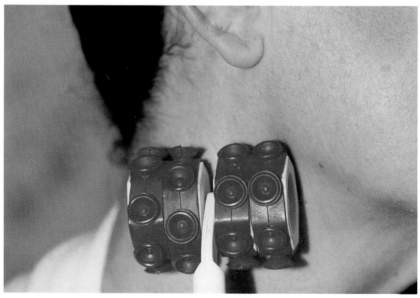

28. Application of the Facial Spirex along the side of the neck to facilitate drainage of the lymphatic system, sore throat, etc.

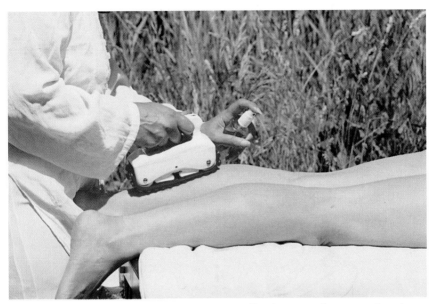

29. Rose-Marie Pénoël demonstrates a Supra Spirex/floral water application on the calves, while stretching the Achilles tendon with pressure exerted by the thigh of the therapist on the foot of the patient. This is excellent after jogging!

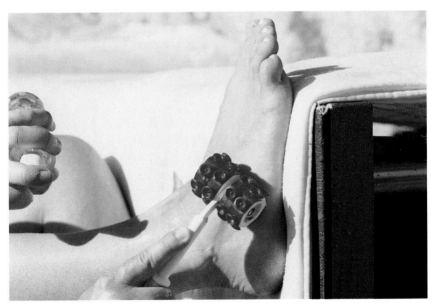

30. Self treatment with Facial Spirex and floral water on a sprain that had remained painful for several weeks. Relief comes very quickly in applications like these.

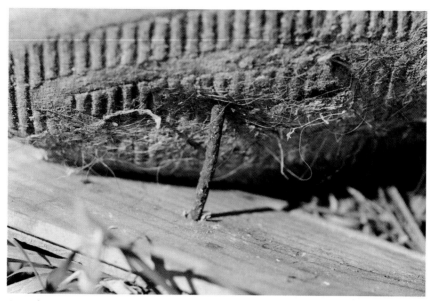

31. This is a close-up of a rusty nail about to pierce through a slipper into the foot. Clearly there are infection potentials from the slipper as well as from the rusty nail.

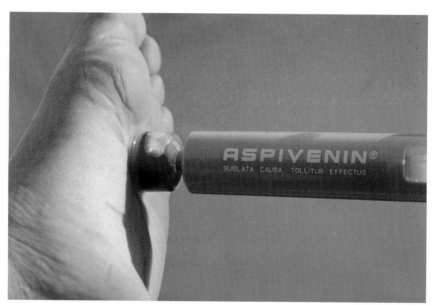

32. Hand pressure alone cannot remove infected blood. A tool like the Aspivenin® (or Extractor®) is required in order to suck out infectious particles. It can be used for puncture wounds as well as snake bites and bee stings.

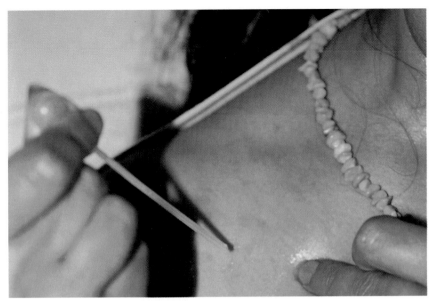

33. Drops of essential oil are applied here on the lung meridian area, just below the clavicle.

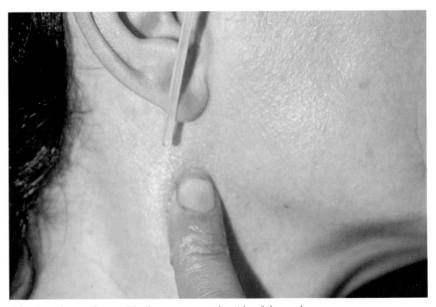

34. Two drops of essential oil penetrate on the side of the neck.

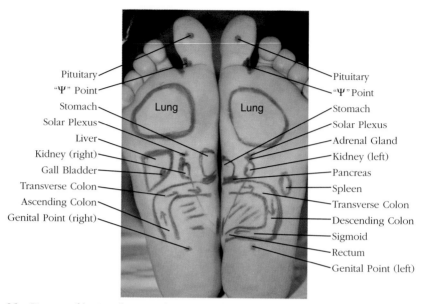

Pituitary
"Ψ" Point
Stomach
Solar Plexus
Liver
Kidney (right)
Gall Bladder
Transverse Colon
Ascending Colon
Genital Point (right)

Lung   Lung

Pituitary
"Ψ" Point
Stomach
Solar Plexus
Adrenal Gland
Kidney (left)
Pancreas
Spleen
Transverse Colon
Descending Colon
Sigmoid
Rectum
Genital Point (left)

35. Diagram of basic reflex areas for the right foot and left foot.

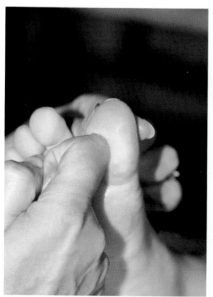

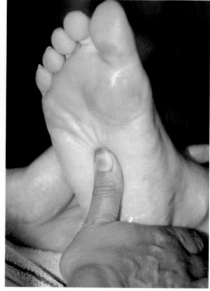

36. Massaging the very important pituitary point with the knuckle of the index finger.

37. Massage of the solar plexus area.

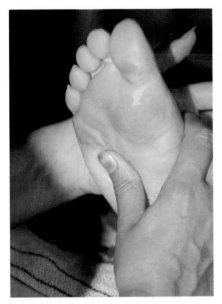

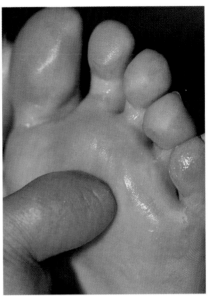

38. Massage of the liver area on the right foot.

39. Massage of the lung area (exists on both feet).

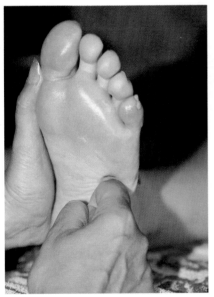

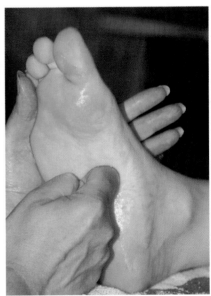

40. Massage of the spleen area on the left foot with index finger knuckle.

41. Massage of the pancreas area on the left foot.

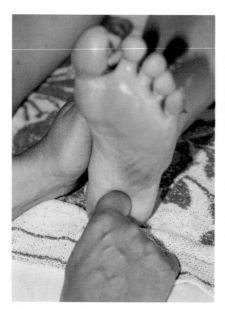

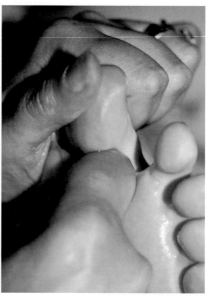

42. Massage of the genital organ area (exists on both feet).

44. Massage of the psi (Ψ) point where psychological trauma accumulates, causing a build up of microcrystals that need to be worked on to "set the spirit free..."

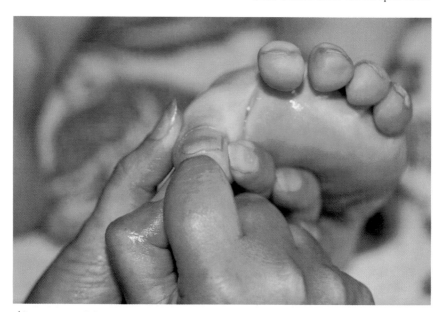

43. Massage of the sinus area on top of the big toe.

– II –

PRACTICAL APPLICATION

ACT

*A*s mentioned in the Preface, Part I was translated directly from the original French version of the book. This second part, however, had to be totally rethought and rewritten for several reasons. The great principles which form the basis of my understanding of life and natural health, as a doctor and a human being, remain the same; but my life is continually transformed by daily discoveries of new ways to apply natural medicine and the growing need for ecological commitment.[17]

My thinking's evolutionary tendency resides in the preponderant role that factors relating to the mental and moral order of things play, or in other words factors that come to play in the psyche and the spirit in general. But that does not change any of the Principles and the Laws discussed earlier. With practice and experience, it is normal for changes, refinements, and improvements to occur. My first duty as a doctor, a writer, and editor is to inform the public and the readers of these developments.

I have structured this second part as follows.

First of all, a chapter focusing on the tremendous challenge of growing and distilling the very highest quality aromatic substances, and cautions on how to find the highest quality essential oils for therapy. Chapter 2 is a "primer" on basic essential oils, including a simple selection of basic, but effective essential oils for regular individual and family use. Chapter 3 includes instructions for using essential oils to handle small emergencies at home and to provide aromatic aid for the total body.

In the context of Abby's story, we have focused on aromatic maintenance for the respiratory system. In this first introductory work on the method, I can't begin to cover all ailments and the care that should be given to all body systems. Likewise, a detailed and complete description of all essential oils and their uses goes far beyond the scope of this book, which remains simple and pragmatic.

Chapter 4 contains descriptions of certain particularly effective techniques that make it possible, for a modest investment, to obtain increased vitality and accelerated results, when used on conjunction with essential oils and floral waters.

In Chapter 5, Rose-Marie gives some nutritional advice and describes certain recipes that played a role in the cleaning and purification process accomplished with Abby. Also in Chapter 5 is an introduction to foot reflexology, as we do it in our clinic, including the presentation of a newly discovered reflex point connected with the mind and emotions. Finally, Rose-Marie presents some valuable direction on proper breathing for better health.

Chapter 6 is a literary question-and-answer session, where I attempt to answer some of the most commonly asked questions at my seminars.

The best way to learn aromatic action is to participate in an introductory seminar, immediately followed by practical application. This intense aromatic experience with all the energy that is generated from an excited and enthusiastic group is an irreplaceable experience, which I would like all my readers to experience someday. These introductory seminars in no way claim to train someone to be a professional aromatherapist, or to take the place of institutes which offer in-depth instruction over a certain number of theoretical and practical course hours. The sole purpose of these seminars is to help a maximum number of people to become more and more responsible in managing their health and more and more independent, which is relatively easy and pleasant, thanks to the essential oils.

For the most difficult cases, nothing can replace the competence of specially trained and highly experienced professionals. For those who cannot participate in these direct training sessions, I have provided in this book sufficiently-detailed explanations, illustrated with actual photographs, to enable you to begin on your own with relative ease and safety.

Are you ready? Then give me your hand and let's start along the road of this exciting voyage of discovery—the discovery of aromatic health the natural way.

CHAPTER 1

THE SEARCH FOR EXCELLENCE
IN ESSENTIAL OILS

"I'd rather have a single drop of genuine essential oil than a 55-gallon drum of junk product."

Dr. Daniel Pénoël

*T*his chapter constitutes a crucial stage in your learning process. It was not written to attack or criticize in a destructive way–although it might seem like it in some places. My only aim is to clearly and simply explain, using meaningful examples and colorful comparisons, what a genuine essential oil should be–and also what it should not be.

I want this issue to be very clear. My first objective in all my medical work is to help build health; it is to heal and eliminate ailments, not maintain them. One thing that is entirely unique about using essential oils in therapy is this: they must be at least "100% pure and natural" in order to have any therapeutic effect. If they are not, they will not heal, and they may even cause unpleasant side effects.

It is a little like the engine in a Formula 1 race car. Such an engine, to work at full capacity, must receive fuel and oil that is appropriate for its high-performance operation. Additionally, it must have special coolant designed to help control the high operating temperatures.

The fuel must be refined to exacting specifications; diesel fuel used in such an engine would ruin it. Likewise, the motor oil used in this high performance engine must be refined to demanding viscosity requirements to control heat from friction. Even the water must not have harsh mineral content, or they will accumulate and block off the channels of the cooling system, putting car and driver in big trouble.

If there is one thing I have seen over and over again in my long career providing care with aromatic extracts, it is that the quality of the therapeutic results is directly proportional to the quality of the aromatic products used.

I do not mean that the quality of the aromatic product is the only condition important for good results, but it is a necessary first condition which must be integrated with other elements in the therapy process.

Let's take a look at the key areas that determine excellence and purity in essential oils.

1. The plant and its growing environment.

Most people who buy a bottle of lavender oil in a retail store do not realize the elaborate chain of events that must take place before that essential oil can be made available for purchase. Nor do they appreciate how frequently essential oils are diluted or adulterated with synthetics and extenders. Nor do they appreciate–unless they have taken the time to study–the dramatic differences in the essential oil production cycle vs. the chemical/pharmaceutical production cycle.

In pharmaceutical production, for example, the raw material most widely used for the synthesis of many medication molecules is petroleum. In aromatic medicine, since the medicating molecules are a product of plant photosynthesis, we are dealing with a non-polluting, renewable resource. When the petroleum resources of the globe are exhausted, Nature will still continue to provide us with plants and their living molecules. In the mean time, a return to the plant world will become an ecological requirement and an industrial reality.[17] I believe the day will come when the earth's inhabitants will look back and say that the age of petrochemistry was a short, but very polluting interlude in the history of mankind.

We find that plant "intelligence" is taken to its highest degree within the realm of aromatic plants–those from which essential oils are extracted. In a future book, I will go into the evolutionary aspects of the aromatic plant world in connection with human evolution. For the moment, however, I want to explain the importance of agriculture on aromatherapy.

To do so, let me use this example: My English-speaking friends love to gaze at the blue-violet lavender fields of Provence. There is something spellbinding about those magnificent natural colors. And yet...what my friends think of as "lavender," pronounced with that English, American, or Australian accent so charming to the French ear (and I believe the reverse is also true) is often not lavender at all, but a hybrid plant–lavandin–which delivers a significantly higher volume of essential oil than true lavender.

But the therapeutic characteristics of lavandin are quite different than those of lavender. This lack of botanical precision is one of the common mistakes made in selecting a high quality essential oil. (We'll talk more about this in just a moment.) But there are additional problems…

When we look more closely at this "lavender" field, we see that among the geometrically aligned rows, hardly a single weed is growing. It is a deception to think that the field grew that way naturally. It is a deception to think that the absence of parasites from these plants is because they have a natural resistance. Unfortunately, it is also a deception to think that these plants are grown the "old way": with organic love and care for the soil.

The most likely scenario is that these fields of lavandin or lavender are cultivated with synthetic chemical fertilizers. They are treated with chemical herbicides to keep the weeds from growing and chemical pesticides to keep pests and parasites down. Why hide the truth? After all, we should be suspicious of any commercially grown product in a world of chemical and genetic folly. This is the reality in a multinational agro-business world, where the primary performance criterion is a maximum of profit in a minimum of time. And those chemicals become part of the plant and can distill out of the plant into the essential oil.

Of course, there is room for some practicality here. If a producer is trying to do nothing more than give a lavender-like scent to a bathroom cleaning liquid or a toilet disinfectant, I am not going to declare war on him for using chemicals on his aromatic plants. But I don't want to hear anyone calling that aromatherapy! And even then, I still have concerns about damage to the ecology and pollution of the soil.

Let's go back the bottle of so-called lavender oil just purchased by a person planning on using it for aromatherapy purposes. Having read about the immense benefits for true lavender oil, as it was cultivated and obtained in the times of Gattefossé, this person, näively but in good faith, is going to use it for therapy as if it was genuine essential oil of true lavender. There is a very strong potential that this person will have some problems with this essential oil, or at the very least, will not experience the expected benefits. This tragedy happens hundreds of times every month: new users, having heard of the potentials for essential oils, go out and buy junk product and when it doesn't work (or creates unwanted side effects), they give up on integral aromatherapy, thinking there is nothing to it.

Hence my motto: "I would rather have one drop of genuine essential oil than a 55-gallon drum of junk product."

With a genuine essential oil of true organic or wild mountain lavender, an application on a cut or a burn will definitely result in a real and observable therapeutic effect. There are several reasons why some so-called "pure essential oils" do not have this desired effect, as follows:

1. Lack of biological precision, i.e. the oil may in fact have been distilled from a related or hybrid plant rather than the plant named on the bottle. (Example: hybrid lavandin is often labeled "lavender.")

2. Chemical pollution due to residues from chemical fertilizers and pesticides used in growing the plants.

3. Loss or destruction of important aromatic molecules due to hasty distillation.

4. Dilution with vegetable oils or synthetic extenders.

5. Adulteration with cheaper essential oils or synthetic chemical compounds.

6. Improper storage, exposing the essential oil to heat, light or oxygen.

Any of the above can neutralize the therapeutic effect of the essential oil, even though the scent still seems normal. I would go so far as to say that still in a majority of cases, unsuspecting people are buying "pure essential oils" that are adulterated. The reason for this is that for decades, the perfume industry put all its emphasis for essential oils on their scent. In English-speaking countries, there was very little awareness of therapeutic action through essential oils until the 1970s.

We have talked specifically about lavender, but the same situation exists generally with all essential oils. We must not be naïve. You must know that greedy manufacturers can go pretty far in this fraudulent activity. For example, it's pretty common–especially in essential oils found in North America–that they have been extended with synthetic excipients. Lavender oil is often diluted and adulterated with the synthetic molecules of linalyl acetate. It is not such a major crime in the perfume industry, and it does occur, because their whole focus is only on scent. When the Japanese do experiments in factories or offices on the psychic influences of fragrances, they diffuse only synthetic molecules into the air conditioning ducts.

Some chemists insist that these synthetic molecules have an "identical nature" to those found in genuine essential oils. But they have never walked in our high mountains of Provence and breathed the spellbinding aroma of a sprig of wild thyme or smelled the delicate fragrance of a flowered head of fine wild lavender. For them, we may as well live on another planet. But I prefer that other planet–real Nature–to their world of artificial fragrances and crude chemical copies.

2. The crucial extraction phase, through distillation or expression.

Not only must we start with the highest quality organic plants in order to obtain therapeutic grade essential oils, but we must also use infinite caution in distilling or expressing the oils from the plants. It doesn't matter how carefully you distill, if the plants you start with are glutted with chemicals. But what a terrible tragedy it is when we start with properly grown plants and then destroy the therapeutic value of their essential oil through a murderous distillation process.

It is like taking all summer to lovingly care for and grow a kitchen garden with gourmet vegetables, filled with life and essential nutrients, and then cooking them in a microwave oven!

Distillation is an almost magical act, an alchemical transformation of life from a mass of solid plant material into a precious liquid substance. Since high heat and pressure can destroy volatile aromatic molecules, it is necessary to lengthen the distillation time, using lower temperatures, to capture the full variety of therapeutic substances that are within the plant. Lavender, for example, must be distilled much longer for therapeutic grade essential oil than would be required for perfume grade essential oil. The lengthening of the distillation cycle is necessary in order to obtain the precious coumarin molecules.

My purpose in this chapter is not to describe all the technical aspects of distillation, but simply to provide an awareness of the various steps in the distillation process and how they affect the quality of the end product. It may be useful to compare the distillation of essential oils with the extraction of food oils from seeds or olives. Let's use sunflower seed oil as an example. In a grocery store I can find refined sunflower oil. It is obtained from sunflower seeds which are grown in a hyper-chemical agriculture system. They are then subjected to a heat-extraction process, aided by petrochemical solvents. They also undergo a multitude of denaturing attacks which, in the end, leave a totally dead product with a longer shelf life. The caliber of this oil is so low, I wouldn't even want to use it to polish my shoes!

If I am willing to pay a higher price, and look harder and go to a health food store, I can buy what is known as "cold-pressed" virgin sunflower seed oil. The seeds for this oil come from plants cultivated according to controlled and certified organic specifications. They are subjected to a mechanical extraction process involving slowly turning presses, without destructive heat. The raw oil is allowed to settle, and is then filtered through paper, and bottled in colored glass for protection. This is the only way plant oils can be extracted with their nutrients intact, making them fit for human or animal consumption.

While I am on the subject of mechanical extraction, I should mention the problems connected with citrus essences. This is a very serious matter. What we call citrus essences are produced from the peels of citrus fruits when they are harvested. Typically, these fruits are raised on large commercial citrus farms which are abundantly sprayed with pesticides. These chemicals accumulate in the peels. The essences are extracted by mechanical presses from these peels. Citrus essential oils often are laden with these chemical residues and therefore are not useable for therapeutic purposes.

I am particularly cautious about the citrus essential oils I use, because they are a pleasant oral medicine, when mixed with a little honey. You must obtain an organic certification for citrus oils, if they are to be used internally at all.[18]

There is now a growing volume of citrus production being cultivated according to organic specifications which will yield essences for therapeutic use. (Sicily now furnishes most of the organic citrus crop for the production of therapeutic citrus essences.)

(Notice that I use the word "essence" rather than essential oil. The reason is that cold pressing yields a product that is molecularly identical to that existing in the peel of the fruit, because it is not altered by heat or water. The word "essence" is used to apply to the aromatic molecules as they are found *in the plant*, or as the result of extraction by expression. In distillation, by contrast, the end product is transformed by water and heat, and so we use the term "essential oil" to make the distinction.)

When I use the term "aromatic substance" I am referring to both the essential oil as well as the aromatic floral water produced in the course of distillation. Floral water is the water remaining in the still after distillation (the essential oils float on top), and it has delightful potentials as an aromatic product, especially if one is geographically close to the distillation location (otherwise, shipping costs for floral water become prohibitive). Floral waters are unique in that they are gentle enough to be used in contact with delicate mucous membranes like the eyes. But here again, because of the way they are used in therapy, one must be especially strict about the organic origin of the plant material in order to avoid problems with chemical residues.

Another type of substance, often confused with essential oils, is called an "absolute." Absolutes can have delightful scents, but they are not essential oils, and they are not appropriate for medical aromatherapy use. The reason is that they are extracted with strong chemical solvents which can be harmful if ingested. Absolutes can be used in English-style aromatherapy, highly diluted for massage or for pure olfactory effect, with relative safety, but should not play a role in any type of aromatic medical care.

I had mentioned earlier the difference between true lavender and hybrid lavender. I want to return to this issue, which is another area of great importance in finding a quality oil.

3. The importance of botanical precision.

This is a much larger problem area than most people realize. To make my point clear, I will use an analogy with cars. Most English-speaking countries would be familiar with the Ford brand in the automotive industry. If you tell a police officer that you saw a wanted man fleeing in a "Ford," his next question will immediately be, "What model of Ford?" There are many models of Ford cars, trucks, and vans, from low-end economy models to high-end luxury models. Even within the same model there are style variations, such as convertible, station wagon, coupe, etc. In the automotive world, it is easy to get lost if you are not precise.

Another example would be trying to find a Mr. Brown or a Mr. Smith in an English telephone directory; or a Herr Müller in a German phonebook; or a Señor Martinez in a Mexican phonebook. Why? Because you will find hundreds of thousands of people answering to the same surname!

In the same way, it is unacceptable in scientific and medical aromatherapy to simply talk about essential oils by using the generic name, that is, using the name of the genus *without including the name of the species*. In fact, it is somewhat of an insult against the aromatic plant world to use generic names, when there is such an overwhelming diversity among and even within the many species.

If you hear or read the words "thyme," "eucalyptus," or "melaleuca," it means practically nothing. In the world of integral aromatherapy, it is too broad to be useful. It is far too generic. Consider this: the name "thyme" does not refer to any particular plant. It is the genus name for a family of plants with at least several dozen different species! Many of those species have several sub-species or varieties and within a sub-species there can exist several different chemical "races" or chemotypes. So you can see that without botanical precision, we could quickly be swimming in confusion.

We have a similar case with "melaleuca," where there are at least a hundred different species belonging to this genus. The situation is even more confusing with the genus "eucalyptus," where we are talking about a vast family with more than 600 different species. If aromatherapy wants to achieve scientific credibility, it must start at the beginning with respect and concern for botanical precision. Allowing imprecision to persist is the same as leaving the door open to fraud and marketing deception of all sorts.

The only way to create this precision is to insist on both genus and species nomenclature, using the system put in place by the Swedish botanist Linné. Going back to my "thyme" example, we would add a species name, such as *Thymus vulgaris* or *Thymus zygis* (a species that grows in Spain) or *Thymus serpyllum*, etc. If the complete double name does not appear on a bottle of essential oil, the manufacturer may not be producing essential oils pure enough for therapeutic purposes.

Even with this level of precision, we may still have difficulty because of variations that exist within species. This takes us into the realm of chemotypes.

4. The importance of chemical precision.

Earlier, I mentioned two Australian chemists, Penfold and Morrisson, who first reported the experience of crushing two identical-appearing leaves from two different trees of the same species of eucalyptus and finding that they did not carry the same aroma. This led them to the discovery of chemical "races" within a single botanical species. In France, sometime later, the Montpellier School of medicinal plants did research which verified the existence of these chemical races, but this time within the species *Thymus vulgaris*. Depending on the predominant molecule type in the essential oil, several chemotypes of common thyme were identified:

Thyme *(Thymus vulgaris)* CT thymol

Thyme *(Thymus vulgaris)* CT carvacrol

(These two chemotypes are irritants because they contain high quantities of phenol molecules. These can burn the skin and the mucous membranes, and must be used with great care. The remaining chemotypes are much milder.)

Thyme *(Thymus vulgaris)* CT geraniol

Thyme *(Thymus vulgaris)* CT thuyanol-4

Thyme *(Thymus vulgaris)* CT linalol

Thyme *(Thymus vulgaris)* CT alpha-terpineol

Thyme *(Thymus vulgaris)* CT terpenyl acetate

Thyme *(Thymus vulgaris)* CT para-cymene

There are eight chemotypes for just one species, *Thymus vulgaris,* and we know that there are dozens of species within the genus, *Thymus.*

In the case of rosemary, we know of at least three chemotypes:

Rosemary *(Rosmarinus officinalis)* camphor (found in Spain and France)

Rosemary *(Rosmarinus officinalis)* verbenon and bornyl acetate (found in Corsica)

Rosemary *(Rosmarinus officinalis)* 1.8 cineole (found in Morocco and Tunisia)

Chemotypical variations do not apply to all aromatic plants, but in those species where they do exist, they must be considered when selecting therapeutic grade essential oils.

Much of the credit for validating and systemizing this botanical and chemical precision in therapeutic essential oils must be given to Pierre Franchomme. During the 13 years of our close collaboration, his scientific approach to precise classification was of constant benefit in my clinical and bacteriological work. Largely due to our mutual efforts, a determined avant-garde trend, oriented toward finding the highest quality plants and essential oils, coupled with a requirement for precision and exactness in using those oils, was created.

Of course, we recognize Dr. Jean Valnet as the one who started the process, but all science evolves. Dr. Valnet did extremely well with what was available to him in his day. But that does not mean that his knowledge and his conclusions are immutable and definitive. If you were responsible for recruiting the most effective engineers for NASA, would you choose engineers from the 1950s who had not continued their education, or would you choose engineers from the 1990s who were up-to-date on the latest discoveries? The answer is obvious.

Let me present a simple scenario that brings all of this home to the world of aromatherapy:

> Two aromatherapy doctors are at the bedside of a young patient, a 3-year old boy with a lung infection which they must treat aromatically. It is found that only two essential oils are available to them. One bottle contains the essential oils of common thyme CT thymol (one that burns), and the other bottle contains the essential oil of common thyme CT linalol (one that is mild, even when applied neat, or undiluted, on the skin). Dr. O (for Old) is from the old school; Dr. N (for New) was trained more recently at a school recognizing the importance and the differences between chemotypes. Dr. N says: "Now, my dear colleague, I know you don't believe in the therapeutic importance of chemotypes, but we must make a choice here, to help this young patient. Which oil shall we use?" Dr. O, despite his old-school orientation, looks at the little boy and knows he must choose in his favor. "Just in case there really is a difference, let's use the milder of these two oils to reduce the risk, if we can, to our little patient."

Can you see how this more current, evolving knowledge is of critical importance in properly treating and healing with essential oils?

The thirteen years of work done by Pierre Franchomme and myself, summarized in our book *L'aromathérapie exactement*, has been the beginning source of precise information for all serious medical aromatherapy work. Pierre provided the excellent botanical research, and I provided the practical clinical and therapeutic applications. Unfortunately, much of that information was exploited by others who had no part in the research, but who claimed it as their own for purely commercial purposes. For this reason, I have concerns about greed and selfishness in the world of aromatherapy.

Is compromise necessary?

In describing this search for excellence in essential oils, I have admittedly described an ideal that is very, very high. This was deliberate. If we do not try to perceive this ideal as possible, we will stagnate in our progress and fall victim to the curse of mediocrity.

The same principle applies in the domain of morality. In a world of violence and degradation where so many around us are willing to cheat, steal, lie, vandalize, pollute, and destroy; if we don't hold up the high ideal, if we don't try to convince others that there is truly another, better way to behave in life, then there is no longer much hope for mankind.

This idealism, however, does not prevent me from being realistic. Let me describe for you the current situation as I see it.

In today's retail mass market, anything can be found. Any extract, lotion, or cream that gives off a fragrance can claim to be "aromatherapeutic." Generally, the chemicals used for fragrancing and flavoring in the commercial market are entirely unfit for therapeutic purposes. More specifically, most of the essential oils available at retail are less than therapeutic grade. The reason is simple: demand and supply. Especially in North America, the demand for fragrancing ingredients is so high and the supply of distillable aromatic plants is so limited, that there is always a market for diluted, extended, and adulterated essential oils. But here again, we fall back into something that should be called "recreational fragrancing." It should never be confused with medical aromatherapy.

If the manufacturers of these mass market lotions, creams, and oils, requested botanical and biochemical precision from their essential oil suppliers, they would find most of them unable and/or unwilling to respond. If it became a requirement, those suppliers would simply move on to other customers who were less demanding. Most of the worldwide "production system" for essential oils today does not fully appreciate or care about the need for therapeutic grade quality.

Even if these manufacturers were able to obtain and use therapeutic grade essential oils, the aromatherapeutic value of their lotions, creams, and oils would still be questionable because the quantities of essential oils used in them are so minute, and generally they are not therapeutic grade. You can begin to see why I use the term, "recreational fragrancing." This is not serious aromatherapy at all.

But times are changing, and new voices are being heard. Several high-level distributors appear to be in a position to provide essential oils that meet extremely strict quality standards, including providing precise classification information on genus, species, chemotype, and growing location. All this makes it possible to know exactly what plants were used in the distillation; exactly how the plant material was distilled and even–in some cases–a complete chemical analysis of the oil as it was distilled. As the world awakens to the true medicinal value of quality essential oils, more acreage will be devoted to organic aromatic crops, and more distillers will begin to distill for medicinal purposes rather than fragrance purposes.

To better illustrate the gradations (or degradations) of essential oils, I can use the example of water. In many places, public water is downright unfit for consumption, because of pollution from chemicals, bacteria, or both. We call water we get from the tap "potable," and it is supposed to be watched and certified by local health authorities. But is it really? We use the same water for drinking that we use to flush our toilets, and the cost for delivering it often dictates a compromise in quality. In order to have a truly good quality of water for human consumption, we need an entirely separate drinking water system. In France–and I think our conditions are somewhat the same as those in other industrialized countries–I encourage my patients a reverse osmosis water filtering system for all their drinking and cooking water requirements.

We can compare water that is potable to the range of essential oils that are intermediate grade. These oils are not acceptable for therapeutic applications. Like potable water, they may be good enough that they will not make you sick, but they certainly won't make you healthy, especially for long-term treatments.

Some Practical Criteria

So where does this leave you, the reader, in finding high quality essential oils? To start with, you should expect and be able to obtain the following information from a prospective supplier:

  – the exact botanical name of the species used in distillation and the
    part of the plant that was distilled or expressed
  – the country of the plant's origin

– the country where distillation took place (myrrh resin collected from trees in Somalia is often shipped to France to be distilled)

– the chemotype of the species, where applicable

– the main molecular constituents through gas chromatograph (GC) analysis

– some indication concerning the organic status of the plants, distinguished as follows:

A. "Conventional Crop" (implying the use of chemical fertilizers, pesticides, and herbicides)

B. "Natural Wild Plants" (which does not necessarily guarantee the absence of chemical residues)

C. "Certified Organic" (meaning cultivated according to organic standards established by an authorized organization)

D. "Conversion Crop" (pertaining to crops cultivated during an interim period while awaiting organic certification)

Anyone can appreciate that essential oils produced according to the above standards will cost significantly more than essential oils that are cut or adulterated to be used in "recreational fragrancing." But there is so much misinformation on essential oils, that price alone does not necessarily give a good indication of quality. One thing is certain, a true high quality essential oil, such as Rose, Lemon Balm, or Frankincense cannot be bought at a bad price!

Remember my motto: "I would rather have a drop of genuine essential oil than a 55-gallon drum of junk product." Quality essential oils are expensive to produce, but they are worth it. If someone offers you a 5 ml bottle of essential oil of rose at a price less than wholesale, there is certainly fraud. Either the pure product has been diluted with some type of vegetable oil (in which case a grease mark will be left when a drop is placed on a piece of paper), or it is a mixture of synthetic fragrances with a small amount of essential oil of rose, or–as sometimes happens–it is simply some other kind of essential oil.

Fortunately, there are some laboratories now working according to standards of quality and total integrity in all the countries of the world. This higher standard of production first appeared in the 1970s with the beginnings of medical aromatherapy, but many old-school producers have avoided these standards because they call into question too many old habits. So almost everywhere in the world, now, there are two approaches to production: one for therapeutic quality, and the other one for recreational fragrancing. Of course, it is up to the producers to choose their own course, but consumers have a right to be informed clearly and honestly about what they are buying. Once all the information is available, each can make his or her own decision with a full knowledge of the facts.

This can be seen in the situation today with Australian *Melaleuca alternifolia* essential oil–commonly referred to as tea tree oil. *Melaleuca alternifolia* is a species that has chemotypical variations. For tea tree oil to be therapeutically valuable, it should consist of about 35-40% terpineol-4 molecules, but also contain a minimum proportion of the 1.8 cineole molecule–usually about 9-10%. An essential oil very rich in terpineol-4, but lacking in 1.8 cineole will not have as well-balanced a healing effect for a therapist using natural aromatic medicine.

On the market today we can find the essential oil of the tea tree produced in three ways:

A. Produced in plantations organically certified

B. Harvested from wild trees

C. Produced on plantations using conventional chemical agriculture

When it comes to making tea tree shampoo or soap, I am not fanatic to the point of requiring certified organic tea tree oil. This is recreational fragrancing. But for intensive medical use, I obviously prefer to have access to certified organic tea tree oil.

Taking practicality one step further, if I must choose between non-organic tea tree oil and an antibiotic, I would choose the non-organic essential oil. This is particularly true if treatment is for an emergency situation and will be of short duration. In contrast, if a patient has been suffering for ten years from systemic candidiasis because of repeated antibiotic treatments, I will choose to wait a few days if necessary, to acquire the organic tea tree oil, because the patient is probably embarking on a treatment that will last up to one year.

I try above all to be logical and practical in my approach. I always keep in mind the ideal situation, the one for which we should be striving. But sometimes that ideal must be tempered by what is possible and feasible.

Conclusion: Patients will determine the future

I am independent of any essential oil production company. I am a teacher and a doctor, seeking to disseminate information which will help doctors and patients alike make good decisions about aromatic health care clear and understandable. I know that, in time, truth will emerge and triumph. My goal is to hasten that day. I am happy to provide my support to any and all who agree to work openly and honestly in the production and distribution of quality essential oils. My personal belief is that it is in the best interests of all producers—and also of the entire biosphere—to orient themselves toward crops which are non-polluting and the most respectful of the entire ecosystem. Aromatic plants fit this requirement perfectly.

The circulation of this English translation alone could have a profound effect on what consumers—the patients of the world—will require from their doctors. I expect many changes in our medical systems in the next 10 years. One of them—and it will certainly happen sooner or later—will be that patients will no longer be satisfied by medical care that costs a fortune and does not deliver results. When medical producers and distributors of all types of products (not just essential oils) realize that a larger, more vocal, and more faithful clientele is turning toward quality natural products, the law of supply and demand will take over—the supply will adjust to address the demand. There are millions of acres of land that require nothing more than to be cultivated properly. There are millions of unemployed people throughout the world who long to take part in a productive life. What has happened in the cultivation of food crops and in livestock farming can also happen in the cultivation of aromatic plants.

In spite of all the changes that remain ahead, I remain confident in the future. I know that many scientists who direct laboratories focusing on aromatic products are seeking more and more to produce their own essential oils, or have them produced at the highest quality levels by investing in existing farms or setting up new enterprises in Third World countries. I cannot complete my mission of informing and training unless— and until—high quality essential oils are produced in abundance for the health and prosperity of everyone. Then and only then will we discover that essential oils can bring us "a wealth of health and a healthy wealth!"

Footnotes

17. In Brazil, cars are starting to run on fuels from sugar cane; in the U.S., several areas are mixing fuel from corn alcohol in gasoline. In France, some buses receive a portion of "green" fuel, so the trend of returning to renewable forms of energy has already begun.

28. If it is a matter of putting a few drops in soapy water to give a citrus scent while washing in the washbasin, I don't require organic certification. But, once again, this kind of application should never be called aromatherapy.

CHAPTER 2

A BASIC SELECTION OF
ESSENTIAL OILS FOR THE HOME
and an
INTRODUCTORY COURSE
FOR THEIR DAILY USE

*I*n Chapter One, we focused on the crucial problem of finding quality aromatic substances, and in doing so, we traveled over a major portion of our journey toward achieving health in a natural, aromatic way. Now we will learn how to put together our own basic aromatic pharmacy. Some laboratories, which I respect highly for their work, have suggested lists of up to 350 different essential oils! This is more for professionals and scientists doing research in aromatic medicine, and in that arena, such lists may be appropriate.

For personal and family aromatic care, however, such lists are impractical. Again, I feel it necessary to state that the purpose of this book is to reach a large, general audience and provide them with simple, practical, and relatively inexpensive ways to safeguard and improve their own health and the health of their families. It is not intended to train eminent researchers in aromacology.

Criteria for my selection of basic essential oils for the home

A long practice of daily family aromatherapy has taught me to understand that in aromatic care, "a little goes a long way." It is far better to understand fifteen or twenty essential oils well and use them daily, than to be lost in an immense, mysterious teeming jungle of hundreds of complex oils.

In Part I, we presented three levels of care:
        –Regular Aromatic Care (RAC)
        –Emergency Aromatic Care (EAC)
        –Intensive Aromatic Care (IAC)

The following criteria were selected not to enable one to address every possible health condition, but rather to get the biggest return for the investment, and to be able to provide effective RAC and EAC. It is something like a mountain climber who must not be overloaded as he starts to climb, but he does want to make sure he has everything essential to the success of his climb.

1. The essential oils should be easily available.

It is particularly disappointing to do exhaustive research on an essential oil and talk about it and write texts praising it, only to find out that the availability of this promising product is ultimately very limited. The essential oils I am recommending have never, in my experience, been in short supply.

2. The products must be able to meet high quality standards.

We will not succeed in obtaining organic certification and therapeutic grade standards on a large variety of essential oils, unless we begin insisting on genuine essential oils and learn enough to avoid and refuse essential oils that have been adulterated or are of dubious quality.

3. The essential oils must be affordable, even in quantities required for daily use.

There may be those rare occasions when we want essential oil of rose or frankincense and are willing to pay the high price required to be sure of getting a genuine product, but for regular aromatic practice involving daily use of essential oils, we want to avoid a financial burden. Buying these oils must not damage the family budget, or regular aromatic care will not be followed very long!

4. The essential oils should be safe to use in almost any circumstance.

This last criterion is one that deserves extensive explanation. There are essential oils that are perfectly natural and that may even be certified 100% organic, but which still entail too much risk to be left in the hands of the general public. Essential oil of pennyroyal mint *(Mentha pulegium)*, for example, is sold freely in the United States, but is a high-risk product. If high-risk oils are allowed on the market too long, sooner or later there will be accidents, and the likely result of that will be intolerable restrictions placed on *all* essential oils. The essential oils recommended here do not include any neurotoxic or excessively irritating varieties.

In a broader sense, however, even when the safest of essential oils are used, there are important precautions that must be followed in any oil application. The next section outlines these guidelines for safe use.

INDISPENSABLE PRECAUTIONS FOR THE
SAFE USE OF ESSENTIAL OILS

This is one of the most important sections in this book. These guidelines must be learned, shared, and consistently practiced, if we want aromatic care to develop and flourish. In every country there have been cases of serious problems, even fatal accidents, resulting from the improper use of essential oils. Most of these problems involve children. Before driving a car, motorcycle, or boat, we must first obtain a license. Learning the precautions described here is like the beginning of the learning process to obtain a license to use essential oils in your home.

Of course, there are drivers (I know several in France) who, once acquiring their license, do not respect the rules they have learned. I hope I can present these rules in a way that will motivate you to always respect and obey them. If you experience a problem in spite of everything, the first two guidelines are intended to counteract emergencies arising out of unintended contact with sensitive skin areas and mucous membranes.

1. Never try to dilute essential oils with water.

As their name implies, essential oils do not mix with water. If they did, they wouldn't float to the surface in a steam distiller, where they can be collected easily by separation flow. So it is important to remember if essential oils should ever irritate sensitive skin, they cannot be diluted with water. Water will cause the oils to burn even more. A comparison can be made to a petroleum fire: water will tend to spread such a fire rather than extinguish it. Essential oils must be diluted with some type of vegetable oil.

2. Never let essential oils come in contact with mucous membranes or sensitive skin.

By the very nature of extraction, essential oils are highly concentrated substances.Essential oils, because of their highly concentrated state, must never come into contact with mucous membranes or sensitive areas of the skin. If so, they should be immediately diluted with a good grade of vegetable oil. My very strong counsel is that a container of vegetable oil should always be included in any kit of essential oils–for safety's sake if for no other reason.

An all-too-frequent case is the following: a person puts a few drops of essential oil on their fingers to rub on the chest or the soles of the feet. This having been done, he or she forgets to rinse the fingers.A few minutes later, with a little bit of essential oils still remaining on the fingers, the person scratches or rubs near the eyes. It is almost certain that this will create some irritation. Other times, and more seriously, a drop of essential oil is accidentally splashed into the eye. In this case, the irritation is very intense. The oil must be diluted immediately. I advise using almond oil if available, which is mildest for the eyes, but any pure vegetable oil will help. Put it on a cotton ball and delicately dab at the eye.

When essential oils come in contact with other areas of sensitive skin (armpits, genital areas, face, etc.), vegetable oil should be applied the same way to dilute the essential oil, thus reducing the irritation.

If essential oil is swallowed, one or two spoonfuls of virgin vegetable oil must be taken immediately to soothe the irritated mucous membranes and dilute the essential oil reaching the stomach. This will also slow down the speed of passage through the gastric mucous membranes and penetration into the blood. For some essential oils, particularly those rich in neurotoxic ketones (officinal sage, thuja, pennyroyal, hyssop),[21] planning should be done to immediately ingest activated plant charcoal, whose adsorption ability makes it possible to stabilize the toxic molecules quickly, limiting their passage into the blood.

3. Never add neet essential oils directly to bathwater.

This precaution must be taken, again, because the oils will not mix with the water but will float on top of it. When essential oils are used this way in a bath, the floating oil will stick to the skin in its concentrated form, particularly to the sensitive genital areas. This can cause a very unpleasant, even serious irritation, because hot bath water actually increases the irritation phenomenon.

Instead, dissolve the oils first in powdered soy milk, egg yolk, or even coarse sea salt. Never try to use more than 10-20 drops of essential oil for one bath. For further safety, add the essential oil/powder mixture slowly over time while you are in the bath, rather than all at once.

4. Generally, people with allergies must be very cautious with essential oils.

My first advice to those with allergies is to choose the very highest quality oils you can find. Residues from chemical agriculture are in fact the most likely source of skin reactions. As much as possible certified 100% organic essential oils should be used. Make a test application by applying a small amount of the essential oil on a small area of sensitive skin. To reduce chances of an allergic reation, essential oils can almost always be applied to the sole of the foot or possibly the areas below the malleolus (on each side of the heel). The essential oils will be absorbed into the body and reach the intended area (generally the respiratory passages) relatively quickly, especially if the skin is warmed first using a hair dryer.

Complete treatment for allergies is a complex subject, not within the scope of this book. I have found, however, that nutritional reform is always required.

5. Some essential oils are light-sensitizing, so exposure to sun must be avoided after application.

This is particularly true of citrus essences, extracted by cold-pressing (expression). The most common case is that of the essence of bergamot, but caution must be used with most citrus oils. Beyond the citrus varieties, I should also mention the essential oils of angelica and African marigold. Ignoring this rule when using these essential oils could result in brown skin patches which could become permanent. There may also be an increased risk of skin cancer.

6. Some essential oils have strong caustic characteristics, and should be used very cautiously, generally in a diluted form.

This applies to the essential oils rich in phenols (thymol, carvacrol, eugenol). Examples include the phenol thymes, oregano, savory, clove, and cinnamon leaf. The essential oil of cinnamon bark (Ceylon or China) is also very irritating. Also the oil of lemongrass, concentrated in citrals, can be highly irritating.

7. Essential oils rich in menthol should not be used close to the throat or neck on children under 30 months of age.

This is the rule taught in medical and pharmacological courses concerning menthol. In natural aromatherapy, we do not use menthol in its pure state, but use instead the essential oil of peppermint, which is very different! Nevertheless, as a supplementary precaution, I prefer to include this rule as it is learned in standard medicine.

8. Care must be taken to tightly close essential oil bottles after use and to always keep them out of reach of children.

This rule is self-evident, but must be restated because it is broken too often. It applies to all chemical products and medications. But I stress its importance for essential oils because there are those who would viciously attack aromatherapy in the event of an accident with children, seeking to destroy a method that upsets them. Sadly, this same problem occurs every day with standard pharmaceutical products, but the same type of scandal never appears.

9. Taking essential oils orally requires oils of impeccable quality and the direction of a qualified health professional.

This basic precaution does not preclude taking them in diluted form in an appropriate excipient. Even so, problems that arise from taking essential oils internally are generally due to the fact that they were taken in a concentrated state which leads to rapid absorption in the stomach and a very quick passage into the bloodstream. Taking one or two drops of a mild essential oil of high quality, diluted in honey, does not entail any particular risk. It just requires good common sense.

10. Always keep some vegetable oil readily available when using essential oils.

Any essential oil kit must contain a vial of good quality carrier oil.

By following these ten cautionary rules, you will eliminate all risk of encountering a problem in using essential oils. Now we can begin to put together our first collection of essential oils.

A BASIC LIST OF ESSENTIAL OILS FOR HOME HEALTH CARE

1. Melaleuca Alternifolia: your first defense against bacteria and infections.

The famous "tea tree oil" (TTO) is now known throughout the world. Its fame is well-deserved. Personally, I have used it in daily medical treatments for seventeen years. Consistent success with this oil has given me great respect for its healing and protecting properties.

The reader who discovers TTO for the first time while reading this book and who, after opening a first bottle expects to experience an beautiful aroma, will probably be disappointed. The fact is, we are talking about the oldest fight in Nature, the fight against infectious disease. The intention of Nature in giving us anti-infectious aromatic molecules is not to launch us to the seventh heaven of olfactory delight. There are other essential oils for that. The goal here is to help the body in its fight against a bacterial attack. There are essential oils for love and there are essential oils for armed conflict. Melaleuca is a fighting oil. Its tour de force lies in its extraordinary antiseptic power and remarkable anti-infectious activity, while retaining an exceptional mildness. It is absolutely non-aggressive with regard to the mucous membranes.

I think of the Australian pioneers who dedicated their lives to making this tree and its essential oil available to the rest of the world, and I convey my deep gratitude to them, on behalf of the millions of patients who have benefitted and who will yet benefit from their patient and devoted research (See Photo Nos. 8 and 9).

Any doctor or pharmacist who has doubts about the antibacterial value of aromatherapy and needs bacteriological, mycological, or clinical proof can find it in an impressive number of research articles focused on this essential oil. Perhaps no essential oil has been better documented in terms of its antibacterial and anti-infectious activity.

At the very practical, family application level, all that is needed is a simple, first-step, "tea tree oil response." It is one of the safest and most effective ways of controlling and eliminating minor infections. The classic example for using this oil occurs in cases of sore throat, pharyngitis, and other throat infections. Such problems must not be neglected because they can quickly lead to serious complications with certain bacteria (streptococcus, for example).

The secret to success in using TTO for combating sore throats is immediate action. The moment you feel that unpleasant tickle at the back of

your throat, signaling that an inflammation is starting, you must be prepared
to act. Therefore it is necessary to keep with you wherever you go a small
bottle of essential oil. It can be in your purse or briefcase. I have used a small
kit that attaches to my belt. If you are at the office, the factory, a construction
site, or even in school, you will not have time to leave and go get a bottle of
tea tree oil at the health food store. You have to keep working and take care
of yourself with discretion. Again, I cannot emphasize enough, the secret is to
start treatment with tea tree oil at the earliest moment an inflammation is
detected. Let's imagine the following scenario:

Mary, 23 years old, works in an office in Detroit as a
secretary. It is the month of January. She caught a cold when
she went out this morning, and by 11:00 am, she felt soreness
in her throat and it was becoming painful to swallow. Mary
knows very well from past experience how this type of problem evolves in her. Normally, she will spend several hours
with a serious throat infection, which eventually turns into a
fever and significant fatigue. She then visits her general physician who always prescribes antibiotics and several days' rest.

But this time, a new element enters the picture. It happens
that a friend of Mary's, who knows her tendency to catch
colds and sore throats, offered her a small book written by a
French doctor and translated into English introducing her to
family aromatherapy. Since then Mary has kept a small basic
kit of essential oils in her handbag. She is willing to carefully
follow the advice in the book, because the doctor who wrote
it has specialized for more than twenty years in aromatic medicine. She has kept the book with her and it is easy for her to
check on the procedure she should follow, point by point.

Mary takes her little vial of *Melaleuca alternifolia* essential
oil, unscrews the cap, and puts the pad of her little finger on
the opening. She turns the flask over to get a small amount of
essential oil on her finger, and wipes the excess on the edge
of the bottle opening. (A trace is sufficient, and Mary remem-
bers that the calculation made by Dr. Pénoël, using Avogrado's
number, shows that just a trace of this magic substance contains about 4,000 million billion molecules of terpineol-4.

That's 4,000,000,000,000,000,000 molecules!) Mary collects some saliva on her tongue and then applies the pad of her little finger to the upper surface of the tongue. Dr. Pénoël had explained in the book that the smell of tea tree oil was not exactly heavenly, but the taste was tolerable, with a hint of pepper or spice. The trace of essential oil mixes with her saliva and, after about 10 seconds, Mary moves the saliva to the back of her throat, where her tonsils are bathed by the oil and its infection-fighting strength. Then she swallows everything, for she also read that the real origin of a throat infection is often inside the intestinal flora. The pathogens did not leap into her throat as she was crossing the street. Mary also knows that she is paying for the excesses of holiday gastronomic festivities, in particular the chocolates which she loves with an unreasonable passion.

This entire process has taken less than 20 seconds and is not even noticed by her co-workers. Within seconds, Mary is pleasantly surprised to feel a noticeable relief from this first application. This discomfort in her throat is slightly anesthetized, but not in the same way those pills from the drugstore (which contain contact anesthetics) do it.

Now the impression Mary has is one of deep and genuine effectiveness, and not a camouflage accompanied by marketing hype. She feels she is getting at the cause and not just covering symptoms. Mary knows that this treatment is really helping her whole body. Dr. Pénoël explained that the secret to success lies in frequent repetition of this simple application, at very close intervals at first, but spacing them according to the relief felt.

Every minute for ten minutes, Mary applies the trace on her tongue, exactly according to the instructions in the book. Additionally, Mary applies a few drops externally: one drop along each lateral surface of the neck (right side and left side), going down from the mastoid process (behind the ear) to the joint between the sternum and the clavicle. She also places a drop to penetrate below the corner of the lower jaw, on the right and left sides. After these 10 internal applications and the

two external applications–all done in less than 15 minutes–
Mary is really feeling confident about what she is doing,
because she feels an action that is both powerful and mild,
and she senses her energy level rising.

She continues the treatment a little less frequently: every
five minutes, four or five more times, then every ten minutes,
every twenty minutes, etc. Mary notices there is some tension
in her shoulder muscles, and this reminds her that Dr. Pénoël
had also said that essential oil of lavender has relaxing properties. Having followed directions to include a small bottle of
lavender essential oil in her emergency kit, she takes it now
and applies a drop or two to the nape of her neck, massaging
it well, using a downward motion.

Mary's co-worker, Sue, sitting in the next cubicle, smells
Mary's "perfumes" and asks her what she is doing. Mary
explains to her in a few words and shows her the book. Sue,
who loves to help out, agrees to massage Mary's neck for a
few minutes. Finally, Sue asks Mary to lend her the book,
because the idea of managing her own health and that of her
children on a daily basis is of particular interest to her. Mary
will go on a little diet for three days, following the nutritional
advice given in the book (by Dr. Pénoël's wife). The whole
experience has been quite convincing.

Mary realizes her body has found a whole new way to be
cleansed and purified of disease. If she had given in to panic
as before, she would now be in bed, undergoing antibiotic
treatment, and tired for weeks, possibly with relapses. Mary
also knows that she has suffered fungal infections following
antibiotics, and she understands this never occurs when treatment is performed with essential oils!

As for Sue, she returns the book in a week, because she
is very enthusiastic about what she is reading and decides to
purchase her own copy. She is particularly moved by the story
and testimony of a little Australian girl, because she has a seven-
year old daughter, Diana, who seems to be heading down the
same road to some degree. She wants to wants to apply the

book's advice and follow a simple and effective program to solve her daughter's long history of "stuffy, runny nose complicated by otitis." She has decided to acquire the Hydro Floss® system which, in addition to ensuring excellent hygiene of the teeth and gums, enables a mild and in-depth cleansing and purification of the nasal cavities. In time, other co-workers in the office will be made aware of this new aromatic approach.

The good news begins to spread slowly, but surely.

Describing this treatment in the form of a scenario like this, illustrates the treatment clearly enough that anyone could conduct his or her own experiment when a sore throat arises. Above all, remember that you must have the bottle of essential oil immediately available so treatment can start at the first sign of infection. And small doses, repeated frequently, are much more effective than one or two large doses.

I deliberately portrayed this scenario away from home to illustrate how easy it is to use the oils in almost any circumstance and environment.

If a throat infection starts while you are at home, you have additional freedom. You can dilute some tea tree oil with a little natural honey, organic if possible, and sip this aromatized honey or let it dissolve directly on the tongue. Combine four drops of tea tree oil with one tablespoon of honey. Take an amount about the size of a pea. With a large toothpick or chop stick, then suck on it. Essential oil of *Melaleuca alternifolia* does not cause irritation and can be mixed directly into the honey.

Important caution: honey does not have the ability to dampen in any way the aggressiveness of the irritating molecules, such as the phenols. If you want to prepare an aromatic honey with an essential oil of thymol thyme, savory, carvacrol oregano, or even eugenol clove, it is absolutely necessary to first dilute the essential oils with some vegetable oil. Organic hazelnut oil is particularly pleasant for this purpose, or even organic sesame oil. Two to four drops of essential oils should be mixed in 10 ml of the chosen vegetable oil. When these aggressive oils are diluted, the diluted mixture can then be mixed into the organic honey. If a very liquid honey is used, the diluted essential oil mixture may have a tendency to separate over time. It simply needs to be remixed each time it is used.

I mentioned earlier the "tea tree oil response." I contrast this with what I call the "antibiotic response," which is ingrained in doctors and patients alike. The task here is to replace "antibiotic response" thinking with "tea tree oil response" thinking, as a first-step, immediate intervention action. We apply this rule confidently for almost all minor problems within the framework of home treatment (though not for serious cases that require hospitalization).

Again, immediate intervention is the key, as a form of first aid. Nothing precludes requesting medical consultation if, at the end of a few hours of aromatic treatment, there is little or no improvement. In such a situation, the ideal would be to consult a doctor or health professional trained in aromatic medicine, who can instruct in more aggressive natural measures.

For ENT and respiratory infections, digestive infections, urinary infections, genital infections, skin infections, infections of the mouth and gums– whatever the location–essential oil of *Melaleuca alternifolia* will give priceless, quick and effective help, especially if you intervene immediately. Hence the importance of keeping an emergency kit with you at all times.

The following is a true story, which took place during our stay in Australia:

> On a Thursday evening I received a telephone call from a family living in the hills above Adelaide. The mother explained that their four-year old son had the beginnings of a lung infection that seemed quite serious. They had just gone to their family doctor, who examined the child and immediately asked for a chest x-ray. The cough, fever, general condition, clinical examination, and x-ray all confirmed the diagnosis of infection, which led the doctor to the "antibiotic response." He immediately prescribed antibiotic treatment.
>
> This is totally logical in the context of conventional medicine. If you press on the udder of a cow, you won't get orange juice, or even goat's milk, but cow's milk. The doctor who has only taken standard medical training; who has not undertaken research outside conventional medicine can't be expected to do anything but prescribe the medications coming from the chemical/pharmaceutical industry.
>
> The parents had attended a conference on natural medicine during which Abby's case had been presented by her father, Robert, my wife, and I. After hearing that conference, they made a firm decision to sincerely try aromatherapy, using

intensive aromatic care at all three interfaces (skin, respiratory membranes, and digestive membranes).

I strongly emphasize the voluntary nature of their decision. This is a hallmark of natural medicine, because natural medicine, requires much more effort than conventional medicine. It requires much more than opening your mouth three times a day to swallow the latest antibiotic fad! One must get deeply involved and pay the price for one's health through real personal study, discipline, and effort. The spirit of natural medicine, then, is quite different from that of conventional medicine, but what a difference it makes in the results.

Since the health food stores in Adelaide stayed open quite late, I asked the father to go get two bottles of essential oil of *Melaleuca alternifolia*. (At the time, there were no serious guarantees of quality for most essential oils, but I knew that generally, tea tree oil produced and sold in Australia was of a quality good enough for intensive medical aromatherapy treatments.) I also asked the father to go to Julia Towhig, a naturopath who had borrowed from me an aerosol system (Osmobiosol®) I had perfected for intensive treatments. Julia was advised of this by telephone, and agreed to entrust the complete system to this family. They were determined to do everything necessary to find a natural solution for their young child.

The father then returned to the house with the special glassware, stand, air generator, and the bottles of essential oil. This family was resolved to follow my instructions precisely. Honey enriched with the essential oil was prepared and the child sucked and swallowed a small amount of it every five minutes at first. In addition, four to five drops of tea tree oil were applied neat–undiluted–on the soles of each foot at close intervals, and a few drops were placed on his chest. This was done for two hours. Then the child was put to bed under the aerosol apparatus.

This is where the respiratory interface came into play. Nighttime hours are usually pretty useless for administering most intensive care, but they are ideal for penetration through the respiratory interface. This was done by creating a fine mist of the essential oil above the child's face for him to breathe during sleep.

The next morning I received a telephone call from the parents telling me that the child had made spectacular improvement. It would be necessary to continue the treatment regularly for three days, progressively spacing the doses and applications. This experience turned out to be a complete success, once again proving the validity of the aromatic method, provided high quality essential oils are used, good equipment is available, and above all, there is a driving motivation to come through no matter how much effort is required.

Aromatic medicine is there to help anyone, but it is not for the lazy and lukewarm. An interesting element of this story is the fact that this treatment was based exclusively on the essential oil of tea tree, thus confirming its extraordinary anti-infectious power, coupled with excellent acceptance by the body, creating no irritation of any kind. Through *Melaleuca alternifolia,* Australia has given the biosphere and mankind a gift of inestimable value.

2. Essential oils from the Eucalyptus family and other essential oils rich in 1.8 cineole: Solutions for clear and healthy breathing.

The next oil I recommend is really a family or rather a generic group of oils. The Eucalyptus genus has many members, and Australia again, is blessed with a climate that favors them. What these various Eucalyptus oils have in common is the 1.8 cineole molecule. To really understand essential oils, we need a knowledge of their molecular constituents and the actions of those constituents. Those who have seen me teach a seminar know that I travel with drill bits. Everyone knows that you can't make a hole in brick, concrete, wood, metal, ceramics, or glass with just one kind of drill bit. Specific adaptation is needed in the drill bit, its alloys, the shape of its point, and the angle of attack in its turns. It is the same, in a scientific and molecular approach, with essential oils. Tens of thousands of aromatic molecules are grouped into large categories according to their chemical functions.

These chemical functions largely correspond to their therapeutic capacity. Some generalization is possible and desirable, particularly from an educational point of view, in identifying therapeutic action with chemical constituents.

For assisting the respiratory function, or more precisely the ventilation function (inhaling and exhaling), Nature has created a molecule whose name itself is significant: 1.8 cineole. *Cine* from the Greek *kine*, expresses movement, and *eol* relates to the wind. In the body, this "wind in motion" is pulmonary ventilation, or breathing.

So in our molecular approach to aromatherapy, we want to choose essential oils containing a significant amount of this molecule, previously called eucalyptol because it was first found abundantly in the leaves of many species belonging to the genus Eucalyptus.

The essential oils I have recommended from this 1.8 cineole group belong to eight different genuses:

1. From the Eucalyptus genus:

Eucalyptus globulus with two main subspecies

Eucalyptus globulus ssp globulus, which is the reference point

Eucalyptus globulus ssp maidenii

Eucalyptus radiata

Eucalyptus smithii

Eucalyptus polybractea CT cineole

There are many other species containing 1.8 cineole, but the ones above are relatively easy to obtain in high quality. Other varieties rich in 1.8 cineole are:

2. In the Melaleuca genus:

Melaleuca cajuputi (or cajeput)

Melaleuca quinquenervia (or niaouli)

Melaleuca linariifolia (CT cineole)

Melaleuca uncinata

Melaleuca ericifolia (linalool and cineole)

3. In the genus Cinnamomum:

Ravensara aromatica

4. In the Rosmarinus genus:

1.8 cineole rosemary (officinal rosemary and pyramidal rosemary)

5. In the genus Lavandula:

Lavandula latifolia CT cineoleifera (spike lavender grown in France; not the Spanish one)

6. In the genus Salvia:

Salvia lavandulifolia (from Spain), provided the chosen CT contains little or no sabinyl acetate

Salvia fructicosa (containing ketones, particularly camphor, so it must be used with caution)

7. In the genus Thymus:

Thymus mastichina (This plant is often known in English as "Spanish marjoram," although it has nothing in common with true marjoram, *Organum majorana.)*

8. In the genus Myrtus:

Myrtus communis (myrtle coming from France, called "green essential oil of myrtle")

Myrtus communis CT myrtenyl acetate (coming from Morocco and Tunisia, called "red or orange essential oil of myrtle")

To understand the genus Eucalyptus, it is helpful to know something about the general world market for essential oils. The largest essential oil-producing country, China, is also the largest producer of essential oil of *Eucalyptus globulus.* Whenever you buy an essential oil of Eucalyptus, there is a strong probability that it came from China. In spite of the distance and transportation expense, production costs in China are unbeatable compared to Western countries.

In general, the Eucalyptus essential oils that appear at retail are almost colorless, while the raw essential oil of Eucalyptus is normally yellow. This is because the retail essential oil is subjected to an operation called rectification or redistillation, which removes certain components. So the essential oil is still 100% pure and 100% natural, but it cannot be labeled 100% "whole." The problem with the essential oil of raw *Eucalyptus globulus* is that it contains compounds that irritate the respiratory mucous membranes, isovaleric aldehyde in particular. An essential oil intended to aid breathing that actually causes irritation and coughing is unacceptable. This problem is corrected through the rectification process, and is an example of human beings acting intelligently.[19]

Spain, where large amounts of essential oil of *Eucalyptus globulus* are also produced, prohibits the sale of the raw essential oil because of the compounds that irritate the respiratory passages. On the other hand, the essential oil of *Eucalyptus globulus* produced in Portugal is sold in the raw state.

Here is a direct, living demonstration of the issue:

As I am writing these lines, I have a flask of raw essential oil of eucalyptus in front of me. It is certified organic, not rectified, and comes from Portugal, and in fact, it is yellow. If I bring the bottle very close to my nose and sniff, I easily recognize the typical odor of crumbled eucalyptus leaves. But I immediately sense a certain suffocation and irritation in the trachea and the bronchial tubes. I also feel a painful impression in my head. If I push the experiment further by placing a few drops on hot (not boiling!) water and breathing the vapors, I start to cough after two seconds and I immediately interrupt the experiment.

Anyone can do this test and feel the same effects. It is not an individual reaction related to a particular condition, but a form of protection on the part of the body. If this experiment is done by a person having asthmatic tendencies, you can expect the start of an asthma attack following this assault on the hypersensitive mucous membranes of the lungs.

If you want to use a whole or raw essential oil, I strongly advise against using it in a concentrated state for direct breathing (on a handkerchief, inhaled, in aerosols, etc.). It is better to use either a rectified essential oil, with the irritating compounds removed, or another essential oil rich in 1.8 cineole that does not contain compounds that irritate the respiratory passages.

The raw essential oil of *Eucalyptus globulus* does have therapeutic potential, but other interfaces (penetration methods) must be used, always with caution and in relatively weak dilutions.

Another essential oil of *Eucalyptus globulus* is produced in Corsica, and is also raw. It is of very high quality (labeled as Demeter or biodynamic, it represents the height of organic production). Its direct respiratory impact produces the same phenomenon of irritation and therefore, it must also be used another way.

This said, from a purely olfactory point of view, we must recognize that there is a fineness and a genuineness in raw essential oil that is lost in the rectified version.

The essential oils of *Eucalyptus polybractea CT cineole*, as produced in the Australian bush in the raw state, is not suitable for direct concentrated respiratory use; the same is true for the essential oil of *Eucalyptus smithii* after the first distillation. Essential oil of *Eucalyptus radiata* normally doesn't need rectification, because it does not contain irritating aldehydes.

Raw essential oils containing compounds that are irritating to the nose and respiratory system must not be used except under certain carefully-controlled conditions. In principle, a whole (or raw) essential oil is the first choice for high-quality aromatherapy. But principles should not be so rigid as to compromise the health or the welfare of the user, especially if the ingredients in the raw essential oil compromise its therapeutic effectiveness.

Nature shows an intelligence that amazes us. But Nature has a universal plan of action, and it doesn't necessarily favor human beings. Molecular aromatic compounds irritating to the bronchial mucous membrane by direct volatile penetration certainly have a role to play from a botanical and biochemical point of view, in the tree's life plan and in the ecosystem, but apparently it is not a role that contributes to human respiratory well-being (at least not in its concentrated form in close contact with the respiratory interface).

Our duty in using essential oils is always *primum, non nocere* [First, do no harm], to adopt the Hippocratic motto. Here's an extreme example: when bitter almonds or apricot pits are distilled, a raw essential oil is produced that contains a lethal compound, prussic acid. It would be absurd and even criminal, knowing this situation, to put this raw essential oil on the market. The only essential oil from bitter almonds that can be found says clearly "FFPA," that is, "free from prussic acid."

In another less-extreme example, when you want to create great aromatic pleasure, you obtain the form of essential oil of Ylang Ylang called "extra." This is the essential oil collected in only the very first part of the distillation process, the part that has the most extraordinary olfactory impact. If my primary goal is to provide an incomparable whiff of exotic escape, I would not hesitate to use the "extra" form, even though it may be incomplete. It's as if the distillation process were split, and the "extra" part is obtained at the very beginning of the process. There is nothing wrong with this choice, because even therapeutic usage recognizes the importance of the sensuous aspects of aromatherapy. So, respect for pleasure plays an undeniable role that is especially important in the olfactory approach and in aromatic massage for purposes of relaxation and well-being.

To my knowledge, there are few texts that pay much attention to these subtle details, which seem to me to be of real importance for a complete, enlightened, and responsible aromatherapy.[20]

In practice, you might argue that the average aromatherapist will mainly find only the rectified essential oil of *Eucalyptus globulus* on the market, anyway. This is true today. But the situation will likely change over time, and some laboratories are already proposing quite a varied list of essential oils of Eucalyptus, including raw ones. Finally, this book will be made available to my Australian friends, who are in a good position to obtain many essential oils of Eucalyptus, even in the "rawest" state. Therefore, my first responsibility as a teacher and therapist is to explain what can be done and what should not be done.

From a practical point of view, here is my proposal for the safe use of raw essential oils of Eucalyptus with cineole, containing irritating compounds:

First, these essential oils must not be used close to the chest in their concentrated form.

Second, these essential oils must not come into contact with the respiratory mucous membranes in the nose or respiratory system. Therefore, I strongly advise against breathing them on a handkerchief, in aerosol, or by inhaling of any kind.

Third, they should only be used in their raw form according to the English method, that is, diluted in a vegetable oil for massage of the body.

Fourth, they can be used in their concentrated state (neat) in the form of a few drops placed on the soles of the feet, or in the form of one drop applied on an acupuncture point.

Fifth, one or two drops of raw essential oil can be taken diluted in honey or in the form of suppositories.

These guidelines allow each therapist to act according to his/her intended objectives. We are focusing on aromatic medicine and complete aromatherapy of a clinical nature, and not purely English-style aromatherapy. Nevertheless, this information guides therapists practicing the English method so they, too, will be able to make essential oil choices in total safety. My summary advice on the subject is as follows:

I recommend having both types of essential oils available. For example, the raw essential oil of *Eucalyptus globulus* (preferably certified organic) in a diluted state, coming from Portugal, is better to use for body massage and perhaps in "aromapuncture." On the other hand, when you need a bottle of essential oil for inhalation over hot water, for the good of your patient please avoid the raw essential oil and use the rectified essential oil of eucalyptus instead (the kind you would find anyway in most stores). Another solution is to choose another essential oil that is rich in 1.8 cineole and lacking in volatile compounds irritating to the respiratory mucous membranes.[21]

The world of the eucalyptuses is a source of fascinating and almost inexhaustible research. When the eucalyptuses grow in areas other than the Australian continent, quantitative and qualitative modifications appear in the composition of their essences.

For some species of Eucalyptus, analysis of the raw essential oil reveals a drop in the level of 1.8 cineole to 50%, and the appearance of some unusual chemical compounds. While these compounds are fascinating to an "enlightened" aromatherapist, they are atypical, so the essential oils would be declared as non-complying when their composition is measured against standard parameters set by official organizations (the AFNOR standards, in particular). But just as the 1.8 cineole molecule was found to have profound therapeutic properties[22] (antibacterial, anti-fungal, and anti-virus), it would be a pity not to investigate the potential contributions of other molecules, even those that occur in lesser amounts. Since rectification eliminates both the irritating aldehydes AND a large number of other precious molecules that appear in trace amounts, you will probably eventually want to obtain a complete raw essential oil of Eucalyptus and respect the precautions outlined previously.

The question of rectification does not come up with the essential oils from other cineole-rich essential oils, because they do not contain these volatile cough-inducing compounds.

One therapeutic quality essential oil that is easily available is taken from the leaves of the Cajeput. The most common source for this essential oil is

Vietnam, but it also comes from Indonesia. The essential oil of *Melaleuca cajuputii* can be used in its raw state. Its price is quite affordable. It is not produced in quantities as large as the essential oil of *Eucalyptus globulus,* but for the present aromatherapy market, the supply is sufficient.

Through distillation of their leaves, other species of the genus *Melaleuca* provide essential oils rich in 1.8 cineole. Most come from Australia. The production cost is higher and the yield smaller, so the price is higher. Personally, I greatly appreciate the fineness of these essential oils, their less "violent," less penetrating, and less aggressive characteristics. In the interface approach developed in integrated aromatic medicine, these mild essential oils with cineole have priority for the respiratory interface, particularly for a constant directional aerosol application (See Osmobiosol® in Chapter Four).

All the 1.8 cineole essential oils play an important role in making breathing easier and in clearing the respiratory passages in general, even at the upper level (nose and sinus).

Nature does things well, from all viewpoints, even on the economic level. The less abundantly an essential oil is produced, the more expensive it is. But when the quality is good, its therapeutic action is so deep and so powerful that it can be used effectively in very small quantities.

For children, and particularly for treatment of allergies, I highly recommend the essential oil of Niaouli (*Melaleuca quinquenervia CT cineole/ viridiflorol*). The one found most frequently comes from Madagascar. It has a slightly greasy feel, or at least it is more viscous then the essential oils of Eucalyptus or Cajeput. In fact, its content of viridiflorol, sesquiterpenic alcohol, can reach 15%. Since viridiflorol has some estrogen-like properties, young women who have a tendency to have short menstrual cycles and abundant flow should be cautious. There is no risk of irritating the respiratory mucous membranes with the essential oil of Niaouli.

An essential oil that I particularly recommend for the aromatic treatment of young children is one extracted from the leaves of the *Ravensara aromatica*. This tree, from the Lauraceae family, belongs to the genus *Cinnamomum* and grows on the island of Madagascar. Its Malagasy name "ravintsara" means "good leaf," referring to the benefits the natives get from it. The essential oil is totally non-aggressive and can even be used close to the face and neck without any problem. In aerosol form, it can be breathed very close to the outlet of the glassware. It can be taken by mouth, and diluted in a good honey, without any problem. For sensitive people who feel the essential oils of Eucalyptus are too harsh for their lungs, the essential oil of *Ravensara aromatica* is a better choice.

Essential oils extracted from the leaves of the common myrtle, while less rich in 1.8 cineole, are mild and very well accepted. The essential oil of myrtle from France is a fairly rare product. It is valuable and expensive, and should be used sparingly.

The orange or red essential oil of myrtle (containing myrtenyl acetate) is produced in much larger quantities. It is often used by smokers in respiratory treatments. It is easy to understand that smokers often experience an aversion, even a repulsion, to essential oils of eucalyptus with a high concentration of 1.8 cineole. Since their system has been literally poisoned, it rejects the very thing that their body most needs to be cleansed and purified. On the other hand, the essential oil of common myrtle, with a lower 1.8 cineole concentration and rich in other molecular compounds, can be used for respiratory treatments for smokers, starting with skin applications.

This essential oil is also used a lot in massaging the spaces between the ribs to relieve areas of tension. Starting next to the spinal column, follow the intercostal paths outward as far as possible. Start at the first spaces and go down progressively to the last. For asthma patients, this is a fundamental aromatic treatment and should be taught to patients so they can continue it at home between sessions.

As for the essential oil of *Rosmarinus officinalis,* the one produced in Morocco is the lowest in camphor. The one produced in Tunisia contains a little more camphor, but both are acceptable. Both are readily used for respiratory and ENT treatment, alone or synergistically. Rosemary from Spain and rosemary from France provide the essential oils richest in camphor, used more for muscle massages. The essential oil of pyramidal rosemary (Rosmarinus pyramidalis) is interesting because it is very mild and weak in camphor.

This book does not aim to develop each essential oil in depth. For the moment we will keep our approach quite general, giving priority to respiratory treatment. In the next chapter, I will describe some quick-penetration techniques often used with the cineole essential oils.

3. Essential Oil of Peppermint (Mentha Piperita): Pain relief and healthy stimulation for the entire body.

Now I want to talk about an essential oil that should definitely be included in your aromatic collection from the beginning: peppermint.

The example of the 1.8 cineole molecule helps us understand the value and need for the molecular approach to aromatic therapy. The important thing for a therapist is first to have the active molecule he needs available. In selecting the essential oils he will use, the therapist takes the following into consideration: the percentage of this molecule in the different essential oils on hand, the molecules synergistically accompanying the therapeutic action of this primary molecule, the possible presence of moderating molecules, and the presence and percentage of irritating or aggressive molecules or even potentially toxic molecules.

Nature designed the 1.8 cineole for the respiratory function and put it in different families, different genuses, and different species. This molecule is obtained from plants growing in different climates, from the subtropics to the temperate zone.

Another molecule invented by Nature that is of major therapeutic importance and plays an absolutely irreplaceable role, is the molecule menthol. Nature put this molecule in two species belonging to a single genus. It is the genus *Mentha*.

In the hottest regions of the planet, the best-adapted species is *Mentha arvensis* (Cornmint), with a high menthol concentration (therefore very "cooling," which makes sense for these hot areas of the globe). For the temperate and even colder areas of the planet, Nature grows another species, *Mentha piperita* (peppermint), which can contains much lower levels of menthol (there are different varieties differentiated by their menthol content).

For medical aromatherapy use, it is best to choose an essential oil of peppermint rather than field mint (cornmint), which is mainly used for industrial extraction of menthol (through refrigeration, the menthol crystallizes and separates). The main action of menthol is to achieve a cooling effect, and even a sense of chilling or freezing, if it is used in the concentrated state. In French pharmacies we find "menthol sticks" to apply on painful areas. In aromatherapy it is preferable to use an essential oil containing additional compounds to balance, synergize, and moderate, all being harmoniously symbiotic.

The quality of the essential oils of peppermint varies greatly. The United States is the largest producer in the world, but the therapeutic criterion does not weigh heavily on such a large market. As a simple flavoring in chewing gum, candy, or even cigarettes, no one can require a certified organic essential oil

On the other hand, for therapeutic use we must be ready to pay more for a product offering the most guarantees. At the production level, organic essential oil generally costs three to four times more than essential oil from large agro-industrial production.

Peppermint is subject to various diseases (rust in particular) requiring chemical treatment. A responsible aromatherapist chooses a "clean" essential oil appropriate to the treatment he is giving. If you want to stop the pain from a blow, with very localized use, it is difficult to require "certified organic" immediately. It is better to use a non-certified essential oil of peppermint and stop the pain quickly than to do nothing because you don't have an organic version of the product with you.

Another interesting aspect is the variation in production areas for peppermint. Peppermint can be made to grow in a broad range of latitudes. From England to Italy, the climatic variation is very great. Qualitatively, peppermint growing in a colder climate will be better than the same plant picked in a hotter country. Extending this comparison, we could say that it may be better to have non-organic essential oil of good quality coming from a colder climate than an organic essential oil growing at a lower latitude.

The hotter climate can cause the plant to create less-desirable compounds (such as pulegone and menthofuran) in larger amounts. If the mint is grown at a high altitude, this factor compensates for the lower latitude. Be aware of the complexity of the situation and all the different factors that come into play in aromatic production for therapeutic purposes.

In a typical household, essential oil of peppermint can play a key role. These are its most important uses:

Pain relief:

Essential oil of peppermint is used mainly to stop pain caused by a hit or blow in a limited area. For example, a blow to the shin, a hit on the hand or foot, fingers shut in the door, etc. The essential oil must be used immediately, hence the concern for putting together an aromatic emergency kit that can be with you at all times. If possible, each member of the family should have one to take everywhere (even on airplanes–we have often had occasion to provide service "in the sky"). It is not necessary to dilute the essential oil for the usual areas of the body (I'm not talking here about a blow to the private parts, where it is out of the question to apply an essential oil neat). If there is also a cut or sore, at least the pain should be stopped by applying the essential oil around the area that is bleeding.

In general, a single application brings remarkable relief very quickly. It can be repeated two or three times if necessary, always in small, light strokes (be careful never to rub the eyelid or touch the eye afterwards with the essential oil of mint on the fingers).

A little anecdote: I had just finished giving my "Intensive internal use of essential oils" class, which includes a demonstration of the use of the aromatic emergency kit.

This happened in England, in September of 1997. Before going on to the second level of teaching we had a day off, so Rose-Marie and I decided to visit Leicester, especially the Indian quarter of the city. As we walked down the main street, an Indian mother and her daughter about ten years old crossed the street. The child happily started running as she approached the sidewalk where we were. Unfortunately she tripped and fell headlong to the ground. Her hand was scraped and in pain, as was her face. She yelled and cried. What could we do? It is hard to remain indifferent to suffering, especially when we know that we are carrying the simplest and most effective way to immediately remedy the situation. Rose-Marie went up to the mother and asked her if she would let us help the little girl with a little essential oil. Distraught, the mother agreed, as did the child. I took the bottle (containing 2 ml) of essential oil of peppermint. I put a trace on my little finger and lightly stroked the injured areas of the face. A few light applications were enough to relieve the pain, and I did the same thing on her hand. The tears stopped very quickly and a shy smile appeared and lit up the girl's beautiful face. What a joy to be able to give effective and natural help so quickly and easily!

The application of essential oil of peppermint, with its anti-trauma action, makes it possible to "create cold" in a way, even in the middle of the road or on vacation in the heat of the summer. This result is spectacular in itself. Once the pain has stopped or been relieved, other aromatic applications are possible and desirable to prevent or treat bruises. The most highly recommended essential oil for this purpose is that of *Helichrysum italicum* (Italian everlasting). I recommend having a small flask of it available to massage the area hit, once the pain is eased by the peppermint. Since this essential oil is rare and valuable, at least one application of high-quality essential oil of true lavender should also be used.

An additional treatment, to be done when you have returned home, is the use of spirexotherapy, complemented by aromatic clay poultices. This will be discussed in the next chapter.

Headaches:

When a headache is coming on, essential oil of peppermint should be applied by small strokes on the forehead, on the temples, and behind the ears. It is not an in-depth treatment, but it helps relieve the pain. You should also massage the nape of the neck, going down from the occipital bone to the trapezium (it is best to also use the essential oil of true or hybrid lavender).[23]

For nausea or motion sickness:

Sometimes it is enough just to breathe a little essential oil of peppermint to stop the nausea. If not, a trace on the tongue or with honey (on a sugar cube if necessary, but in general it is best to avoid sugar) will allow it to work more effectively.

For digestive problems:

Essential oil of peppermint acts quickly and well on all the "hollow" organs–stomach, intestines, and gall bladder. It works particularly well to calm painful spasms. For difficult digestion, overeating, or stomach discomfort, it facilitates the passage of food taken in excess or in the wrong combinations. This is no reason to repeat the same mistakes, but for occasional use it is good to be able to rely on such a faithful and devoted friend as the essential oil of peppermint!

For a stuffy nose:

When the nostrils are very congested, you can't breathe the essential oils through the nose; nothing gets through. So I advise preparing honey with essential oil of peppermint. Put three drops on two tablespoons of good honey, not too liquid. Mix the aromatic honey well and put an amount the size of a pea on the tongue. The volatile molecules will go behind the pharynx and into the nasal cavities, decongesting them and opening up the passage. Try this technique before an aerosol treatment. If you want to obtain a longer-lasting action, I advise obtaining a good honey, organic if possible, sold in honeycombs from a beekeeper or a specialty store. The aromatized honey with essential oil of peppermint is added to the honey in a piece of honeycomb and you can take enough to make a natural chewing gum.

For temporary fatigue or lack of energy:

Essential oil of peppermint is a remarkable stimulant for the entire organism. It revitalizes the functioning of organs, activates the psycho-neuro-hormonal and sexual system, and revives and sustains physical as well as intellectual work. Therefore you should avoid using it before going to sleep. Don't try to cheat Nature by subjecting your organism to an exhausting schedule and then asking the essential oils to fix everything! But for occasional use in the context of a reasonable lifestyle, it is good to be able to rely on essential oil of peppermint!

For hiccups:

Here is a trick that has often worked to stop hiccups. A trace of peppermint is put on the finger and then on both sides of the fifth cervical vertebra. To find it quickly, touch the large vertebra at the base of the neck; this is the first dorsal vertebra. Then go up three notches to find the fifth cervical vertebra. Just put the essential oil on each side of the vertebra without trying to massage, and the hiccups will stop in a very short time (from one second to one minute).

4. Essential oils of true lavender and hybrid lavender (lavandin): Nature's burn medication and stress reliever.

The Drôme, the French county that is first in production of aromatic and medicinal plants, is often called "the cradle of lavender."

A high-quality essential oil of true lavender is an irreplaceable gift of Nature because it provides so many benefits. Unfortunately, large-scale production has forgotten the tradition of respect and the sense of sacredness for this plant and its essential oil. In the fragrancing industry it must be produced fast and cheap and sold fast and cheap, so this amazing aromatic substance has been reduced to an industrial commodity, used primarily in adulterated form for recreational fragrancing.

I have already made mention of lavender and its hybrids and the production methods involved. Therefore, I want to be very clear that genuine results require using very high-quality products. If not, the depth of the disappointment felt will be proportional to the mediocrity of the product used. The essential oil of a hybrid lavender grown organically is more valuable than an essential oil of true lavender of inferior or dubious quality.

In the mountains of Provence, the people use lavender for all sorts of problems, pains, sores, burns, bruises, bites, stings, spasms, etc. Like a reflex, they have acquired an immediate response. We might call it the "lavender bottle response" which is similar to the "tea tree oil response" It has become a part of their culture because they always have a bottle of essential oil of lavender on hand.

True mountain lavender, called fine lavender when it is picked in the wild state, distilled at low pressure for a long enough period of time (up to 90 minutes), produces an essential oil that is incomparable in its mildness, its inimitable fragrance, and its therapeutic qualities. In the context of household aromatic care, both emergency treatment and daily hygiene, here are some indications for its use:

For burns:

Let's think about the experience of Gattefossé and his burned hand immediately immersed in the container of essential oil of true lavender (of high quality at the time). The application of essential oil of true lavender–as long as it is genuine and of high quality–is one of the most effective immediate responses for burns. This said, other essential oils are also very effective, including the essential oil of Melaleuca alternifolia, in particular.

There is a good synergy in mixing them, for example 2/3 or 3/4 essential oil of tea tree to 1/3 or 1/4 essential oil of true lavender. Generally (not just for burns), this Franco-Australian aromatic marriage increases the power of each essential oil over what it would be when used separately. This is not for treating extensive or deep burns, but a response for everyday first and second-degree burns occurring in the home. Another complementary oil for treating burns is obtained by soaking St. John's wort in a good, organic virgin olive oil.

In France, many natural medicine enthusiasts have adopted the "green-clay poultice" reflex, which is very effective for local treatment of burns. A small amount of essential oil can be included to obtain a synergistic effect.

To calm and relax:

The molecular pair present in essential oil of lavender is linalool/lynalyl acetate. These molecules have well-known calming and sedative properties. Therefore the essential oil of lavender is recommended for nighttime use to promote release of the stress accumulated during the work day. The best way to use it is the diluted massage, as taught in English-style aromatherapy. Five drops of essential oil of true lavender in 20 ml of vegetable oil for a local or general massage provides well-being and relaxation.

The main area to relax, if you don't have time to massage the entire body, is the nape of the neck and the shoulders.

For respiratory and ENT treatment:

Infection fighting is not a main function of the essential oil of true lavender. When more effective weapons are available (like *Melaleuca alternifolia*) its role becomes complementary. For example, in the case of a cough with spasms, it is used in association with respiratory and anti-infectious essential oils to relieve the spasms. In the case of otitis, to ease the pain, one drop in the concentrated state is gently massaged around the ear. Or ten drops of essential oil of *Melaleuca alternifolia* can be mixed with 10 drops of essential oil of *Ravensara aromatica* and then five drops of essential oil of true lavender. A small drop of this mixture can be applied around the ear every minute for the first five minutes. In an acute case, you must act very quickly using the oil blend neat.

If essential oil of hybrid lavender (lavandin) is chosen, there are several varieties. The one that comes closest to the essential oil of true lavender is called "super," and it is rich in lynalyl acetate. The essential oil of the lavender hybrid Reydovan, rich in linalool, takes priority for anti-infectious treatment.

The essential oil of the lavender hybrid Abrial contains a little more camphor and should be used cautiously, especially with children. Finally, the essential oil of spike lavender (*Lavandula latifolia*) is used mainly in synergistic respiratory blends.

5. Essential oil of tropical basil: an effective antispasmodic for the digestive tract.

In France, selling the essential oils of anise, fennel, or star anise–which can, under certain conditions, work as antispasmodics–to the public is prohibited by law. These essential oils all contain anethole, a molecule of the ether family with anti-spasmodic properties. Therefore we have gotten into the habit of using an essential oil that is affordably priced and readily available, extracted from the leaves of tropical basil (*Ocimum basilicum, CT methyl chavicol*). When spasms occur at the abdominal or even gynecological level, apply this essential oil locally, in external massages, for easy and fast relief. For the stomach, put a drop on a spoonful of honey and dilute it in hot water. This makes an herbal tea that is very pleasant to drink and aids digestion.

When a girl complains of uterine cramps during menstruation, a few drops of essential oil of tropical basil can be applied to the lower abdomen. You can also use essential oil of taragon, similar in composition in relation to the methyl chavicol. A very typical essential oil which gives good results in this case is that of clary sage (as opposed to officinal sage, a very different plant!).

6. Essential oil of geranium (*Pelargonium x asperum or graveolens*): for wounds to the body and soul.

There are many species and varieties within the genus Pelargonium, and an entire book could be written on this rich and complex botanical world. My main intention in the specific context of this first book is only to propose an essential oil that is easily usable for cuts and open sores. The particular interest of essential oil of geranium is first to facilitate bleeding, which cleanses the wound of possible infecting particles, and second, to contribute to coagulation and the beginning of healing.

When a cut occurs, for example, on the finger (still in the category of small, non-dangerous sores), put a few drops of essential oil of geranium on some cotton and put the cotton on the cut, applying pressure for one minute. Then cover the cotton with cling film and put a bandage over it. Change the bandage after twelve hours, and you will already see some tissue repair.

The essential oil of Rock Rose *(CIstus landaniferus)* has good hemostatic properties, but it is more rare and more expensive. For general family aromatherapy, I like to recommend essential oils that are more readily available and reasonably priced at the high quality level.

Essential oil of geranium is widely used in massages for relaxation, always diluted in vegetable oil, either alone or in synergy with complementary essential oils. It is soothing and relaxing, therefore it Is generally used for nighttime massages for practical reasons. It has a great many properties which aromatherapy books in the English language explain in detail (this essential oil with a strong fragrance is used less in the more medically-oriented French aromatherapy). Its impact on the mental and spiritual realms is largely recognized and it also helps bring harmony on the physical and the physiological level. This psychosomatic perspective is an important part of aromatherapy practice.

This completes my recommendations for a beginning aromatic care kit for the home. With this first aromatic collection, you can address most of life's everyday health problems within your family.

Other essential oils will be discussed in the next chapter on applications and treatments coupled with techniques. I have deliberately limited the number of essential oils to those that I recommend including in the intervention kit. For a reasonable investment, every family interested in aromatherapy can have one or several kits on hand.

You will need to add a flask of high quality vegetable oil as a protection and remedy against contact on sensitive areas. For eye irritations, I recommended including a small flask of aromatic floral water of organic Roman chamomile. You just have to put a little bit on some cotton and apply it on the irritated eye to relieve little eye or eyelid irritations.
Complementary oils advised are the following:
  macerated oil St. John's wort (burns)
  macerated oil of calendula (wound healing, scar tissue)
  macerated oil of arnica (bruises)
  oil of calophylle inophylle (cold pressed), used mainly on cold sores,

with a little essential oil of niaouli and of ravensara aromatica. As for the green clay, it is most practical to have it in the form of a ready-to-use paste, for example, in a tube prepared by the laboratory or in a closed glass container prepared at home.

This basic investment will enable you to provide great service to yourself, your family, and your friends who are open to this aromatic message.

7. Australian Rosalina Oil: the latest aromatic gift of Australia to the aromatic world.

At the beginning of this list of essential oils, I mentioned that the genus Melaleuca comprises many different species. We discussed the amazing anti-infectious, anti-bacterial, and antifungal properties of the alternifolia species, and how it is a highly versatile essential oil for both intensive aromatic care and daily aromatic practice. Now, in a more clinically-oriented vein, I am happy to present officially a brand new essential oil from the Melaleuca family, being launched worldwide exactly at the time of the publishing of this book in the English version. This is just another example of the synchronicity of events which fills all our lives. The tree from which Rosalina oil is distilled is called *Melaleuca ericifolia* (family of the Myrtaceae) and it grows in northern New South Wales.

The leaves and terminal branchlets of the privately managed natural trees are cut and steam distilled. Aromatherapists will love to work with it and to use it with their clients, especially in the context of ESA, i.e. diluting the EO in a carrier vegetable oil to give body massage. This is not because the EO is strong or irritating; on the contrary, it is exceptionally gentle, even when applied neat on the skin. It is simply that using it in a diluted massage is the way to obtain its maximum benefits. When studying a new EO, it is important to analyze the subject from three points of view, which are related to the Aromatic Triad presented in Part I.

The "matter" aspect starts from the understanding of the molecular components, qualitatively and quantitatively. In short: what are the different aromatic molecules and what are their relative proportions? Here we reproduce the data provided by the company who produces Rosalina oil:

Significant constituents	R₁	Area%	Range%
α-pinene	4.790	7.6	5-10
ρ-cymene	6.870	2.4	1.0-4.0
limonene	6.970	2.8	1.5-5.0
1.8 cineole	7.107	23.3	18-26
γ-terpinene	7.813	2.6	1.5-4.0
terpinolene	8.670	3.4	2.0-5.0
linalool	9.335	48.6	35-55
terpinen-4-ol	11.450	0.8	0.5-3.5
α-terpineol	11.943	1.9	1.5-4.0
aromadendrene	19.718	1.1	1.5-4.0
viridiflorene	21.504	0.8	0.5-3.0

Once we have this list of constituents, we get a confirmation of what our nose perceives: we have a very good balance between three major aromatic molecular families...

Alcohols: linalool, a-terpineol, terpinen-4-ol (41.5% to 62.5%)

Oxydes: 1.8 cineole (18 to 26%)

Mono- and Sesquiterpenes (with no oxygen in the structure):

a-pinene, para-cymene, limonene, (γ-terpinene, terpinolene, aromadendrene, viridiflorene (13% to 35%)

It is important to notice the relative proportions of the constituents. In this case, the prevailing molecule is linalool (35-55%). We are dealing with natural biochemistry of plants, not with a synthetic industrial production; therefore, we must accept the fact that variations exist. This is the way Nature functions, even if chemists and pharmacists complain about this fact. Our choice is to work intelligently with Nature; we understand the unavoidable differences from one crop to another. For Rosalina oil, which will be used rather for its energetic and subtle influence, this variability will not create any serious concerns. A holistic approach to essential oils and aromatherapy helps us understand that, though molecular knowledge has its relevant place, there is much more in an essential oil than just chemical constituents. If this were not true, we could simply mix together the synthetic molecules issued from oil chemistry and claim that what we have done is identical to Nature. This, again, is chemical craziness.

You should remember that this analysis of the Rosalina oil shows only the significant constituents and that there are many more molecules than the eleven quoted above. From a biochemical point of view, we know that alcohols have good anti-infectious and especially antibacterial properties. Because of the significant presence of 1.8 cineole, we can deduct that Rosalina oil will be helpful in treating the respiratory system, especially for infections of the upper respiratory system. This is because it is so mild on the skin that it can be applied two or three drops at a time along the side of the neck (on the area of the lymphatic nodes).

For children who are prone to ENT infections, like Abby was, Rosalina oil is a good choice, either by itself or in a synergistic blend that will reinforce its action. In fact, Rosalina oil reminds me somewhat of the essential oil of *Thymus mastichina* (commonly known as "Spanish marjoram"); but in that case 1.8 cineolee content (50-75%) is higher and linalool content (10-20%) is lower. And *Thymus mastichina* is an EO that I often use for treating children with ENT infections. It is a good idea to create a Spanish-Australian marriage by blending both EOs in balanced proportions in order to increase their impact on the mucous membranes.

Make sure that you get a high quality "Spanish marjoram" EO, especially if you intend to use it with infants and children. Organically certified *Thymus mastichina* EO is a bit more expensive, but the high quality EO that you get is worth the investment. The skin is the best interface for Rosalina Oil. Because it is a very new EO, we will collect more information in the coming months from aromatherapists who use it. But I think it is important to provide some basic guidelines and then to gather the results of each therapist.

Whenever you work with a new EO, if you want to experiment in a more "scientific" manner, it is better to use it by itself in the beginning. If used blended with other EOs, it will be difficult to obscure its intrinsic properties and specific actions. After enough data have been collected relating to this new EO, we will have a better understanding of what to expect from it, by itself. At that point, it makes sense to begin to create synergistic blends using it, based on its components as well as on its observed results.

From the Energy point of view, the high content in linalool accounts for its deeply relaxing effect. Linalool is considered a molecule which is soothing to the nerves, calming and even to a certain degree sleep-inducing (hypnotic). For this reason, Rosalina oil should be used in the evening or even before going to sleep. Unless other dynamic activities are intended in bed, Rosalina oil massaged in the back will quickly trigger a state of letting go of the tensions and induce a deep sleep. The good thing is that this Yin action is harmonious and respects the body and the brain. When you wake up, you do not feel like a person who is taking pharmaceutical sleeping pills

Rosalina oil should be applied in the English way. There is no use, from the Energy medicine point of view, to utilize high concentrations, as it will not give better results, We find again the law of "more is less" which is rather surprising for a mechanically-trained Western mind, and, on the contrary, quite easy to grasp for the Oriental mind.

Readers who are professional aromatherapists, will want to introduce Rosalina oil in their practice. It will be perfectly suited for the whole body massage, from the toes to the crown of the head, including massage of the face since it is so gentle on the skin. Here again, it is important at the beginning to use it by itself. For a whole body massage, you can dilute about ten drops in 30 milliliters of carrier oil. This is an average concentration. It can range from 5 drops to 15 drops. Mind you, I am thinking here in French drops (we count with a pipette that delivers smaller drops) and if you let the EO directly out from the vial through the included dropper, you would put 5 to 7 drops in 30 ml of carrier oil.

It is important to know that your patient or client might fall asleep on the massage couch after the session. Therefore, you should allow a certain time for her/him to relax quietly before receiving the next client (the best arrangement being to have two work rooms). For the respiratory interface, Rosalina oil is superb when diffused with the Osmobiosol®, having the outlet directly facing the nostrils, using a very low output of air (if your pump has a regulator, it is very easy to find the right air flow). Again, it will be highly sedative. A patient who comes to me under stress, in particular with strong and accelerated heartbeats and an arterial pressure that appears excessive, would immensely benefit from a full session, with the aromatic massage followed by a complementary rest under the Osmobiosol®. Ideally, this is the kind of treatment that should be available in integral aromatherapy care centers. Of course, make sure your patient does not have to rush out afterwards for a hectic busy day. This kind of session is adapted for after work, for relaxation, or on a day off.

From the strictly olfactive information side, Rosalina Oil is quite interesting to analyze in all its subtlety. Now, I want to pinpoint a factor that seems of major importance to me, after so much time spent with EOs. When you discover and analyze a new EO in a seminar where you will smell it briefly on a testing paper, there is no possibility to perform a serious work.

The "olfactive-respiratory" approach to a new EO should be done in conditions of meditation or reverence (the best French word is "recueillement") you gather all your senses and your psychic capacities to "make one" with the very essence of this tree and receive an inspired message from it). This is a procedure to do when you are alone at home, the phone being disconnected and the children (and spouse) out of your home, so that you have at least the favorable material conditions to undertake this inner travel accompanied by your "new aromatic friend."

The "centers of action" of Rosalina Oil are definitely the upper ones, from the heart Chakra to the throat and the third eye. However, it should be remembered that many problems existing in the lower sphere (solar plexus, navel, hara, root chakra), particularly with human beings, are immensely influenced by disturbances and blockages in "upper spheres." This is one of the reasons for a holistic choice of action, which is much different from the allopathic reductionist approach. Integral aromatherapy is able to focus on local or regional problems, without forgetting to replace them in a wider context, in which the psyche and the body are in constant and intense interdependent relationship. Though there are no esters or ether molecules (for direct antispasmodic action) in Rosalina oil, because of its profound nerve- and mind-relaxing effect, it can work indirectly on the digestive area which is so closely related with our state of mind and our emotions.

In the holistic approach, which is best suited for Rosalina oil, the full or partial body massage, if performed by the right person in the right context, will enable the essential oil to work at the best of its subtle healing and balancing potentialities. Its gentle fragrance will surround the patient and the skin penetration of a small amount will work on many different aspects of the body, from its physical aspect to its finer, hidden levels.

In France, we have access to a chemotype of thyme *(Thymus vulgaris)* which is very precious and expensive: it is the linalool chemotype. I am not saying that Rosalina oil is the same as this one. However, since Rosalina oil will be produced in larger amounts and for a more affordable price than the French common Thyme CT linalool, I simply suggest that therapists do more research in comparing these two oils and see what the results are. In the first place, Rosalina oil will be tested separately and the results will be carefully monitored. In a second place, it might be interesting to blend 90 or 95% of Rosalina oil with 10 to 5% of common thyme linalool chemotype. This would create a powerful yet subtle synergy while remaining easily affordable. Given the strains on today's family budget, we need to be sensitive to the financial aspects of using essential oils.

You should remember that the authentic EO of *Thymus vulgaris* linalool CT cannot be purchased at a low price (if so, be careful; it cannot be a genuine undiluted EO). The subtle balance of cineole (which remains in a lower proportion) associated with linalool and nicely accompanied by well-balanced hydro-carbonated molecules should make Rosalina oil a staple one for in-depth treatments of children known in homeopathy as having a phosphoric constitution and a tuberculinic terrain. Those children are rather thin, nervous, easily infected; they are intelligent but highly sensitive and they react excessively to their environment. In particular, if conflicts exist within the family, they will feel them with abnormal intensity and develop inner problems that allopathic drugs do not address. In order to provide these in-depth treatments, I suggest that Rosalina oil be used over at least three periods of three weeks, interrupted by one week off. The best way in that case is to talk with the child and explain to her/him that every night, when she/he goes to bed, mom or dad will come with a nicely perfumed natural oil to give a very gentle massage on the back followed by an even more gentle massage on the tummy, on the breast and around the neck. Then, she/he will receive a kiss and fall asleep for an aromatic night! When it comes to working on the psyche, I have stated that this "before sleep" application exerts a wonderful influence. Of course, this massage approach does not prevent us from trying to find a solution if a conflict exists between the parents! And maybe this new aromatic attention paid to the child every evening, one day mom, next day father, will help to trigger a new dialogue between the partners? At least, this is my deepest wish.

I leave you now discovering your new aromatic friend and I am sure that all of us together, united by the same feeling of deep respect and love for this latest immigrant in the aromatherapy world, will work for a better understanding of its healing, prevention and personal development potential.

And let us collectively give thanks once more for this Australian essential oil gift, sent to us by the continent blessed by the aromatic gods...and the dedicated workers who extracted Rosalina Oil.

Dr. Daniel Pénoël, Drôme Valley, July 3rd 1998

Footnotes:
19. In his classic book *AROMATHÉRAPIÉ*, Dr. Valnet tells of a friend who had applied a composition containing the essential oil of Eucalyptus globulus, and then saw an asthma attack start immediately afterwards. This friend then explained that every time he went by an area where eucalyptus trees were growing, he had to take a long detour to prevent an asthma attack.

20. There are some very valuable reference books in the English language. From a technical and toxicological point of view, the book by Robert Tisserand and Tony Balacs, *Essential Oil Safety* (Churchill Livingstone, 1995), represents a great work of gathering scientific data. Many other books unfortunately appear to be copies of copies of copies!

21. The detailed descriptions and the advice for differential use of the raw or rectified essential oils of Eucalyptus have not yet been discussed in detail in the books currently available. My position as a total medical aromatherapy practitioner, combined with my position of responsibility as a consultant for laboratory production and work, allow me for the first time to tackle and clarify this subject.

22. Tony Balacs has made a very detailed study–"Cineole-rich Eucalyptus" in *International Journal of Aromatherapy (1* 997, vol. 8, No. 2). Although the failure to mention the irritating aspect of certain raw essential oils is regrettable, the article is very complete and its conclusion is the following:

"I would rather celebrate these wonderful products of nature and use them responsibly than ban them; in skilled hands they are safe, therapeutic substances which are an important part of the aromatherapist's medicine chest."

23. When the headache starts at home, here is a recipe that has often worked: cut a potato into slices 3/8" thick- put them end to end on a cloth or napkin folded into quarters to make a pack a little wider than the forehead.

Put the forehead on the potato slices by lying on the pack and wrapping it around the forehead and temples to the back of the head. Lie down awhile with this "poultice" in place. Very often, the headache is greatly diminished by this simple and natural procedure. In any case, you should think about massaging the nape of the neck (going down) and relaxing the tense areas at the occipital bones by rotary massages.

CHAPTER 3

PRACTICAL AROMATIC TREATMENTS:
Daily Maintenance and Intensive Treatments
for Vibrant Health and Well-being

he purpose of this chapter is to propose and explain a number of treatments and a few complementary techniques, focusing on respiratory tract and ENT problems. These treatments and techniques have been proven over twenty years of medical aromatherapy and clinical practice. I know their therapeutic value and how easy they are to apply.

In this first book, I have chosen to present those treatments that can be applied in the office of a physician or naturopath without expensive, heavy equipment and without lengthy training. These treatments are easily learned and can be continued at home, once the objectives and methods are well understood by the patient. It should be clear that the complete program applied to treat Abby, by contrast, included more elaborate techniques involving specialized equipment.

Some basic support systems are presented in the next chapter. More elaborate technological systems exists, and their presentation will be included in future publications. But we must start at the beginning. As therapists and families alike learn these basic procedures, a great deal of progress in health will be made.

I want to present more of the framework within which these treatments were developed. Clinical and medical aromatherapy requires a different approach, a different mentality, than diluted aromatherapy (ESA) does, especially for anti-stress and psycho-olfactory purposes.

I would like, first of all, to go back to the most important differences that exist between these two principal systems. In order to make these necessary differences well understood, I shall use several comparisons. The first analogy concerns walking and running.

The most natural way to get about is to walk. We might amble slowly, walk at normal speed, pick up a fast pace, or even race walk as in competition. Nevertheless, all these are examples of walking. As soon as we advance to a jog, the muscles and movements are different from those of walking. It is the same for a horse speeding up from a walk to a trot: there is a fundamental change in the type of motion.

When we decide to participate in a fitness program such as one that might accompany a diet, walking or jogging may be preferred. What is one of the great differences between the two? It is this: To burn the same number of calories, we must walk four times longer than we must jog. For example, instead of 30 minutes of jogging, we would have to walk for two hours! This "calorie-burning" aspect is a mathematical part of the comparison. In fact, jogging also influences respiration, the heart, the mind and will, internal balance, etc., in ways that walking cannot. Even walking fast fails to create the same effect as jogging. We must recognize and accept that there is a difference in the fundamental nature of these two types of exercise. In our daily living, we normally walk; for exercise, we run or jog. For our purposes, this exercise comparison applies as follows:

A. The English aromatherapy method corresponds to walking;
B. The proposed method of medical aromatherapy corresponds to running, and even sprinting.

Indeed, let us place ourselves in the framework of physical exertion, but in a situation that involves high risk. Imagine that during a walk in the mountains, a female boar ran from the bushes and, believing its young to be in danger, began to chase us as fast as she can go. Obviously, with no weapons to protect ourselves, we will react immediately in an instinct of self-preservation. Do you think we will run away casually like the joggers we see on the street each morning? No, it is a matter of run or die! We have no other alternative than to run as fast as we can to avoid being torn apart by the boar.

In French we say that "fear sprouts wings," and this is so real that even with a physical ailment like a sprained ankle, our brain will secrete the necessary chemicals that will erase the pain momentarily to aid us in our flight. "English-style Aromatherapy" (ESA), normally requires no urgency or intensive effort. Walking–the diluted aromatherapy as it were–allows the desired result–stress relief and calming–to come to us with relatively little effort. In the context of medical treatments, especially for disease and infection, we are obliged to take up another style of treatment. Jogging corresponds to regular aromatic care; sprinting to urgent or intensive aromatic care.

Now I want to return to our analogy of running from danger. Imagine a hiker out in the mountains with a net to catch butterflies. In this case the hiker also happens to have a handgun to defend himself. As he walks about looking for butterfly specimens, he stumbles on the same wild boar. She is still mad and charges him at top speed. Do you think that the normally peaceful hiker's first reflex will be to wave his butterfly net at the animal to fend it off? No, he will grab his weapon to defend his life. Clearly, it is necessary to adapt the instrument to the desired result. His handgun is useless in catching butterflies, his net useless in protecting him against wild boars. In each case, the hiker adapts his response to fit the situation. The same is true in aromatic care.

The butterfly net = English Style Aromatherapy.

The handgun = Medical Aromatherapy

(Urgent or Intensive Aromatic Care).

Let me make one more comparison with athletic training, specifically body building through weight-lifting. Imagine athlete #1 attempting to build up his muscles using weights that range from 100 to 1000 grams. Now imagine athlete #2 making the same attempt with weights ranging from 5 to 50 kilograms. Athlete #1 can exercise eight hours a day, seven days a week, but he will never develop the muscles he wants. Why? His weights are too light. At best, he could exercise isolated small muscles like those that work the fingers, but he is not on the road to looking like Arnold Schwarzenegger!

Using the heavier weights, even a half-hour each day, day after day, athlete #2 will build large muscle groups quickly. In much the same way, when we enter the world of medical aromatherapy, we seek to achieve dramatically different results by using heavier doses of essential oils, used in more concentrated forms, especially when they are applied through the skin.

I often use the term "integrated aromatic medicine." Personally, I believe all aromatherapy should be "integrated" in the sense that aromatherapists should have the knowledge and the freedom (and the open-mindedness) to resort to one approach or the other, English Style aroma-therapy or medical aromatherapy, depending on the need and the situation. Learning to catch butterflies on the one hand and knowing how to protect oneself from life-threatening dangers with a defensive weapon on the other, seem to me to be altogether complementary skills.

Enjoying a peaceful walk, jogging, and sprinting each have their own merit and usefulness. To meditate upon the beauties of nature, a peaceful walk is unequaled in opening the eyes to the soul. To strengthen the body and the will, jogging is irreplaceable. To escape danger, sprinting at high speed is an instinctive and sometimes life-saving response.

The problem in aromatherapy arises from the very nature of aromatic substances. Their olfactory and subtle energy aspects have made for the development of soft and soothing aromatherapy, which is wondrous and indispensable in its proper application. The aspect of the strong, concentrated aromatic substance has given birth to clinical and medical aromatherapy, especially against infectious diseases.

The field of love and sexuality provides another analogy, though quite different, between the three principal aromatherapeutic orientations.

A. The purely olfactory approach can be compared to "platonic" love. There is no physical contact and less than a trace of essential oil is sufficient to stimulate the nasal receptors. (Information)

B. Diluted aromatic massage, in this analogy, parallels "sexual" love, but for purely romantic reasons. (Energy)

C. The concentrated and deep application of essential oils used in clinical and medical aromatherapy compares to the ultimate act of penetration to fertilize and create new cells and new life. (Matter)

I hope I have succeeded in illustrating the difference between these approaches. If this book has helped you accept of all the diverse modes of application, then it has already achieved one of its fundamental objectives.

Clarity in these concepts and accuracy in philosophy and intellectual classification seem to me to be of greater value than the mere accumulation of a mass of poorly organized and vague facts. The deeper we probe beneath the surface of things the greater tolerance we have for all forms of aromatherapy. As long as you keep these distinctions and goals well in mind, I can begin describing the applications and techniques without risk of shocking you too much.

The great rules of intensive aromatic therapy

In English Style aromatherapy (sometimes I call it "relaxed aromatherapy") it is necessary to dilute essential oils with vegetable oil. The method involves a light, but unctuous massage of the body and concentrated ("neat") essential oils are not appropriate to such an "anointing."

In ESA, essential oils are not slightly diluted, but *significantly* diluted in the vegetable oil, typically the percentage of essential oil in these mixtures is on the order of 2-3%–sometimes less but generally never more than 5%.

What happens when we use them without diluting them? With many current essential oils, nothing dangerous or serious will happen! The problem is as follows: From the standpoint of subtle **energy** and **information** content, maximum results can be obtained with a dilution of 2 to 3%. In fact, stronger concentrations, usually do not provide stronger treatment; often they are weaker! This phenomenon echoes the well-known holistic adage, "more is less."

In medical aromatherapy and especially within the framework of urgent or intensive treatment, the objective is to get the essential oil to penetrate, with its concentrated material energy (aromatic molecules) into the body. Not only do we want to achieve this penetration of **matter**, but we seek ways to facilitate and accelerate the speed of the penetration. While recognizing the extreme importance of massage and its irreplaceable value in all its aspects, the medical aromatherapist uses all three interfaces to get the aromatic ingredient in concentrated form in urgent combat with infection from bacteria, viruses and fungi.

As soon as essential oil is mixed with vegetable oils, transcutaneous transfer (absorption through the skin) will be slowed. This is the exact opposite of medical aromatherapy's goal to create high-speed penetration.

The following four rules outline the new thinking behind intensive aromatic care:

Rule No. 1: During the intensive combat phase, essential oils are applied and absorbed in their concentrated form (neat) through the skin.

During a complete session of relaxing massage, the quantity of essential oils to be used is about ten drops, sometimes a bit more, but the quantity remains very moderate. And this is just fine. During intensive treatment, the total quantity of aromatic ingredient applied is much greater; the more intense the infectious attack, the more volume of essential oil is used. When a flu virus enters the respiratory system, it multiplies very rapidly inside the cells. Even starting with a single virus (and there are always far more), can quickly multiply into a hundred others, which become ten thousand and then a million and so on. This rapid multiplication explains how we end up, in the space of just a few hours, stuck in bed, stricken with chills and fever, aches and pains, a cough, etc.

Rule No. 2: Faced with an attack from these infinitely small invaders (bacteria, fungi and viruses), the body's natural response is to marshal its own army of infinitely small defenders. The essential oils provide ammunition to these defenders in the form of millions of aromatic molecules. The quantity of concentrated essential oils used has a direct effect on the body's ability to fight back, and it must correspond to the danger of the situation.

A natural extension of this rule is that applications of essential oils should be repeated frequently at first and less frequently thereafter.

Rule No. 3: We strike hard and early, making a "furious attack," and maintain the pressure until we see improvement, then progressively space out the applications.

In order not to cause a skin irritation, we adhere to a "cycle" or switching of the zones where the ingredient is to penetrate.

Rule No. 4: We can utilize different zones of the body by switching each time. In all cases, the zone offering the least risk of irritation is that of the soles of the feet, which can stand up to repeated application.

These are the principal rules of cutaneous (skin) application of essential oils in intensive aromatherapeutic care. These rules have been applied thousands of times and have allowed us to solve often difficult and urgent medical circumstances. It is always necessary to use good sense and to understand that what attacks the body leaves us no choice. We tend by our nature to be peaceful, but how can we ensure peace in the face of infectious aggression? By immediately counter-attacking in such a way as to eliminate all attackers as soon as possible!

At a workshop given in Los Angeles in 1991, I stood before two hundred aromatherapists from all over the world, but all were trained in the "relaxed" English method. My goal was in fact to make them understand what I call "the way of the Aromatic Warrior."

I spotted an aromatherapist in the middle of the room who did not radiate health and fitness. I asked her to come up and speak about herself, and she accepted willingly. She explained to the gathering that she had suffered a flu infection in January (the conference was in early May) which was complicated by bronchitis and a permanent infection of all the respiratory tracts. Her family physician had "bombarded" her with the usual antibiotics and other classical remedies, but the results were mixed.

When I discover such a condition in a patient, I am not pleased at all. But to witness such a state in an aromatherapist, who is armed with the weapons necessary to get herself out of this state, made me uneasy. She should have counter-attacked immediately and, with her aromatherapeutic training, cut off, amputated, and torn out that infection! With proper essential oils, if this aromatherapist had received correct information and the right training, she would have known how to react (and even prevent) the first signs of attack and would not have found herself three months later the victim of useless and debilitating medical difficulties.

The lack of information, partial information, or incorrect information leads to paradoxical and very inconvenient situations. Imagine the uncomfortable state of an aromatherapist who must practice his treatments on his own patients while coughing, sneezing; tired out by a lingering infection that has lasted several months! It is understandable that we might find ourselves unprotected momentarily and for a short time even fall ill to a winter infection. But the persistence of this state and its advancement into a chronic one, not to mention the inability to put an end to it (though proven means exist) is what shocks and saddens me and even makes me a little indignant!

In this sort of case, if the patient is willing to provide full support, I apply an intensive treatment according to the rules I have already discussed. At the end of five or ten minutes, a remarkable change comes over a surprised patient who had been "sharing" his or her life with infected mucous and post-nasal drip.

As I have had this experience among "ESA" aromatherapists the world over, I feel completely confident in publicizing this method. The facts speak for themselves! My objective has never been and will never be to cast relaxed aromatherapy in a bad light.

I have such a respect for it that I hope with all my heart that it will succeed in France for the betterment of my compatriots (who happen to hold the absolute world's record for the consumption of tranquilizers!). I am simply saying that if we can agree to supplement the teaching of the "soft" approach with easy, clear instructions about the "hard" method, we will achieve an integral aromatherapy that will give every aromatherapist infinitely greater autonomy and effectiveness.

Example of an ideal intensive aromatherapeutic session

To describe an intensive session, I have chosen an example typical of a winter-time bronchial infection afflicting a patient named Wendy. Initially, the infection is a flu virus, but there is risk that it will quickly develop into a bacterial infection. Wendy, 36, is married to John and the mother of Peter, 13, and Patricia, 11. Wendy calls Betty (her naturopath who has had integral aromatherapy training) and asks if she can come right in for an emergency treatment because she knows that it is necessary to act quickly.

It is 4 pm when the appointment is made and Wendy arrives at 6 pm. She is accompanied by her husband and her son, Peter, who came to learn how to support the treatment at home. Wendy undergoes the first treatment and this treatment will be the opportunity for her to learn how to continue the treatments at home. Wendy in fact shows the symptoms of an infection that is quickly gaining power over her. The medical exam and diagnosis go normally during the first part of the appointment, including an interview to set up the file and the clinical examination. But in aromatic medicine, our medical work has only just started, whereas traditional medicine is finished at this point. Indeed, Wendy will receive an intense aromatic treatment right in the office in order to act quickly against the viral infection and the bacterial infection which typically follows. Since Wendy has had occasional problems with allergic skin reactions, the neat essential oils will be applied primarily on the feet and around the ankles.

The principle of molecular synergy is used in preparing an essential oil blend. Knowing that the treatment is to combat a progressive pulmonary infection accompanied by mucous secretions and an inflammation reaction, it is possible to adapt the treatment to the situation, symptom by symptom. This correspondence between the physiopathological processes that underlie the symptoms and specific types of aromatic molecules allows us to counter-attack vigorously and specifically. This constitutes the molecular basis of aromatic medicine. We analyze the situation and select the oils with the molecular ingredients in the right concentrations to attack the various problems we encounter. Finally, we create synergy by adjusting the proportions of each essential oil in the blend.

In using this scientific approach, we are not tied to a single formula. Botanical and biochemical science allows us a degree of choice, as long as the molecules are present in sufficient quantities. The basic formula in this case, must necessarily contain a large proportion of 1.8 cineole accompanied by a percentage of monoterpenic molecules. In practice, this result is obtained by mixing an essential oil generally of Myrtacee with an essential oil of Conifers. This "marriage" of oils from these two families ensures:

- good respiratory protection
- maintenance of good fluidity of secretions
- genuine antiviral action
- and an aid to the effective penetration of other aromatic molecules into the body.

By way of example, consider this Australian-Canadian basic respiratory formula:

EO of *Eucalyptus radiata* (20 ml)
EO of *Balsam Fir* (4 ml)

This basic formula can be enhanced with additional essential oils to add greater synergy to the blend. Here is the first example of a synergistic formula to add to the basic respiratory formula:

Antibacterial: EO of *Melaleuca alternifolia*: 3 ml (terpineol-4)
Anti-inflammatory: EO of *Eucalyptus citriodora*: 0.5 ml (citronellal)
Loosening mucous: EO of *Eucalyptus dives*: 0.5 ml (piperitone)

And here is a second example of a different synergistic formula to complement the basic respiratory formula:

Antibacterial: EO of *Palmarosa or Monarda fistulosa*: 2 ml (geraniol)
Anti-inflammatory: EO of *Litsea cubeba* (May Chang): 0.5 ml (citrals)
Loosening of mucous: EO of *Carum carvi*: 0.5 ml (*d*-carvone)

The two cetonic molecules that are included in each formula, piperitone *(Eucalyptus dives)* in the first, and carvone (*Carum carvi*) in the second, were selected based on data given by Robert Tisserand and Tony Balacs in their book, *Essential Oil Safety.*[24]

Using this molecular reasoning, it is possible to work out more complex synergies. The important thing is to understand the basic principle, which is the relationship between the physiopathology and the properties of various molecules. Speaking in this molecular language, it is often possible to carry on a productive dialog with a doctor or pharmacist who is open-minded and sincerely interested in understanding and learning.[25]

Aromatic molecular synergy is thus used immediately, within minutes after starting the first appointment, through carefully developed essential oil blends, (limiting ourselves to application only on the skin of the feet in order to avoid any risk of irritation elsewhere on the body.) Once the aromatic molecules enter the body, they are quickly carried toward the organs and, in particular with the cineole vector, they soon reach the lungs and even the mucous membranes of the upper respiratory system, including the ENT region.

In applying the treatment on the sole of the foot, it is best for the sole to be face up and oriented horizontally. Wendy therefore lies face down with a pillow slid under her abdomen to avoid stress to the lumbar vertebrae. Her leg is bent 90 degrees back toward her thigh, in order for her foot to reach a horizontal position (See Photo No. 14). To make the skin easier to penetrate, it is first warmed using a hair dryer to raise the skin temperature (See Photo No. 13). Applying essential oils to cold feet is inefficient and would detract from the treatment, given its urgency. Using a plastic pipette, the essential oil blend is applied in drops, one or two at a time, onto the feet, concentrating first on the pulmonary reflex areas of the feet. For a first dose we want fifteen to twenty drops to penetrate into each foot. The treatment takes two or three minutes. The reflex zones are not massaged *per se,* except to obtain quick penetration into the skin.

I often advise placing a little drop on the tip of the toes between the bottom of the toe and the nail. The sinus points are found there, and the combination of reflexology and aromatherapy creates an excellent synergy (See Photo No. 15). No vegetable oil is used in this case, because it slows penetration. To use vegetable oil here would be like trying to go someplace quickly, but leaving the car's transmission in first or second, instead of fourth or fifth gear.

Once aromatic penetration has been achieved, we can, if we desire, proceed to massage the reflex zones of the foot, in particular the pituitary, hepatic (liver), pancreatic, pulmonary (lungs) and renal (kidneys) areas (See Photo No. 35). This massage is different from the high-speed application used to make the essential oils penetrate. I personally favor this complementary therapeutic treatment. Plantar reflexology is quite well known among the English community (and less well known in France). The problem with doctors is their unwillingness to spend time with their patients. Spending two minutes to help an essential oil blend penetrate into the feet might be acceptable. Spending half an hour doing reflex massage on the feet seems to them to be unreasonable!

In Wendy's case, she will have to continue the treatments on her feet at home. She can also use the sides of her heel under the ankle bones. Her husband, her son or her daughter can help her by following the same approach with the feet. Or, she can administer the treatment on her feet herself. In this case, Wendy sits comfortably on the couch, supported by cushions behind her back. She folds her right leg and brings her foot straight up to rest on the top of her left thigh to bring the sole up as much as possible. After warming her foot with the hair dryer, she rubs in, one by one, about ten drops of the essential oil mixture (See Photo No. 13). She does the same for the left foot. In this intensive phase of the combat, she can perform three applications the first hour—one every twenty minutes. After each application, she drinks a glass of water or, better yet, an infusion prepared from plants especially for respiratory problems. To ensure continuity in the therapy, Wendy will have prepared an aromatic honey, by placing one or two drops of her oil blend in 3 tablespoons of honey. She will use 1 teaspoonful of this honey in a cup of herbal tea.

During the second and third hours, Wendy applies the synergistic oil blend (we call it a "synergy" in France) four times—once every half hour. She observes that she is experiencing distinct progress. She can see that the virus is falling to the counter-attack. When it is possible to begin the battle as soon as the invasion is detected, there is every hope on our side for a rapid and total victory.

Before going to bed, Wendy uses a simple technique that will ensure that the treatment continues during the night. She puts five drops of the synergistic blend on a cotton pad. She applies a "cling film" to hold the pad on the pulmonary zone of her right foot and puts on a sock to hold it all in place. She does the same for her left foot. A few drops are placed on the front and back of her nightshirt or pajamas at chest level. It won't be a romantic night, but it will certainly be an aromatic one that will keep up the fight against her infection.

In general, aromatic "pressure" on the infection must be kept up for several days with the frequency of treatment slowly diminishing as symptoms decline. The results of this method are excellent. By using high-quality products and by observing the retreat of symptoms to adjust the spacing of treatments, there is every likelihood of success. The big risk of all infectious diseases is letting the virus multiply and invade the organism and letting bacteria grow in the mucous membranes of the respiratory system. By using repeated aromatic penetration, the chances of a quick and total healing and cleaning of the body are maximized. This will lead, once the battle is won, to a feeling of purification and a strength much different from the feeble state in which the body is left by conventional treatments.

Afterwards, Wendy will take a daily preventative measure during the heavy winter, which consists of using essential oils to protect the respiratory system. The other members of her family will learn to protect themselves in the same simple and effective manner. In case of alarm, Wendy will know how to act quickly. She has acquired a great deal of self-sufficiency and feels she is in charge of her health and that of her family. She is solving the little afflictions of winter that become big problems if they are neglected or poorly-cared for by a health system that doesn't have the necessary weapons at its disposal.

Having made this overview of the intensive treatment, let's now take a look at the two basic elements in Regular Aromatic Care: the morning tonic and the evening relaxation.

Morning invigoration and evening relaxation: the beginning and end of daily aromatic action

Our concern thus far with the intensive treatment has been to learn to strike hard when infections arise, with the appropriate weapons and munitions, correct strategy, and intelligent tactics. Fortunately, for most of us this disease battle is not a permanent condition! However, for those who live in the stress and pollution of our major cities, there is, in fact, a constant low grade war that our bodies must fight. It isn't wild beasts anymore that we fight in our "struggle for life," but insidious and yet very real enemies.

All the thousands of pollutants breathed or swallowed constitute a constant threat to cells in our body. To this, we can add the hazards of noise, nervous stress, electromagnetic pollution and working at computer screens, psychological trauma caused by news of world catastrophes, emotional conflict at work and at home, and more. This accumulation of several orders of trauma exacts an extraordinary toll on the body and mind.

In the context of natural choices, numerous products and methods abound to help us. It is not my purpose to make a long list of everything available. Each person must choose that which is the most useful and practical in his or her life style.

But I would like to make a few important points about the explosion in the aromatherapy market in products, nutritional supplements and cosmetics.

First, let's look at finances. An average European, American, or Japanese family has a limited budget for matters of health and well-being. By acquiring some essential oils on a modest budget, it is possible to gain great benefit in terms of energy, relaxation, protection, and prevention, at a relatively small cost. A small bottle of good quality essential oil might seem expensive, but if the equivalent health value in plants were purchased instead, the price would be multiplied many times!

By considering both criteria (price and effectiveness), we find that money spent in aromatherapy yields the best investment. We should factor in the value of time, also. With essential oils used according to the techniques proposed, we get rapid results without consecrating an exorbitant amount of time from our active, urban lives.

And last, don't forget the dimension of pleasure and the senses. They are a major plus in the attraction behind aromatherapy that cannot be found in swallowing a gelatin capsule full of nutritional supplements.

My ideal advice is to gather together the greatest possible number of health products and apply the best methods for protection and well-being. My practical advice, considering city life and budgetary constraints, is to develop a habit of "maintenance treatments" with essential oils in daily life.

Such treatments will not replace the work of professionals for serious troubles, but we can still learn to check the oil in the car and add some when the level is down or put gas in it before it runs out, even without seeing the mechanic. For many, it is the "do-it-yourself" formula and for others, the "have-someone-do-it-for-you" formula that is the most attractive. In either case, learn to invigorate your body before going to work and learn to relax from the stresses once back home. These are two pieces of wise advice that are within the grasp of all families. I will outline some simple and inexpensive ways to add these pleasant tasks to your daily life.

For the early-morning invigoration, there are several approaches. The most important thing is to set up good habits that require little time and yet result in good benefits. The morning aromatic treatment can be done while in the shower or just after. By way of example, here is a simple essential oil formula to use that is inexpensive:

EO cajeput: 10 ml

EO Melaleuca alternifolia: 3 ml

EO rosemary with cineole and camphor: 1 ml

EO Picea mariana (black spruce): 1 ml

This formula will open the respiratory passages and lend a psycho-neuro-glandular invigoration to approach the day full of motivation.

One possible application is to turn off the shower, place five drops of this blend in the palm of the hand and spread them quickly onto the chest and extremities. This requires but a few moments, when the skin is warm from the shower. Another possibility is to apply the drops as you leave the shower. Merely wipe away any excess water and spread the drops onto the body and extremities. The still-wet skin has become aromatic and the application can be completed with a loofah glove, tracing the acupuncture meridians up and down the extremities.

For those who are allergic to the blend, it is best to apply it to the arches of the feet. In a sitting position, three to five drops may be placed on the sole then applied by rubbing the two feet together as one would do with his or her palms (See photo No.16). Doing it this way, rinsing the hands isn't even necessary!

In both cases, the objective is to get a small quantity to penetrate very quickly for the purpose of energizing the body and supporting it all day long.

In the evening, we get home full of stress and concerns as well as annoyed by all that went on at work. The minimal treatment that I recommend for evening time is an aromatic massage of at least the back of the neck and the shoulders before dinner. For relaxation massage, here is one example of a synergistic essential oil blend that works wonders to bring relaxation and peace:

EO true lavender or lavendin (super): 4 ml

EO petitgrain bigarade: 1.5 ml

EO geranium: 0.5 ml

EO ylang ylang extra: French = five drops (2.5 English drops)

Now here, the "English" method is a must! It would be useless and wasteful to apply these subtle and energy-rich products, so concentrated in intensive olfactory information, in their pure form. Pour one tablespoon (15 ml) of a good-quality virgin cold-pressed sunflower or sesame oil into a small dish and add two or three drops of the above relaxation blend. This oil will be applied as a soft unction with the fingers on the back of the neck and the shoulders. Start at the occipital processes and go down all the cervical vertebrae and out to the shoulders.

Obviously, this massage may be done using only cold-pressed oils and without the essential oils. Such a massage is in itself a valuable relaxation technique, but two or three drops of essential oils will bring an increase in the relaxation effect that would otherwise be missed. Here again, even with the expense of purchasing essential oils of the best quality, the investment is still quite reasonable, even for regular, daily usage. If desired, one may continue on down the back, after making the person being massaged lie down.

The relaxation blend may also be applied to the solar plexus and the abdomen in order to release any accumulated tension there.

Now that we understand the techniques of intensive treatment and the basic methods of applying daily treatments, we need to learn some supplementary techniques that are valuable not only as treatments or cures, but also as preventative and health-maintaining measures: Hydro Floss®, aerosoltherapy with Osmobiosol®, spirexotherapy and periorbital massage using a glass rod. And we will learn how to use a valuable emergency device, the Extractor® (or Aspivenin®).

Footnotes:

24. This is a good example of French-English complementarity. Prudence is certainly worth more than ever for a family of molecules that includes some highly toxic representatives! It is now appropriate to reestablish a more delicate balance by analyzing, molecule by molecule, the risks or absence of risks. Piperitone and carvone, according to the work presented in the valuable manual, seem to offer a very great margin of safety.

25. To carry on a dialog with an inconsistent or hypocritical partner, in bad faith, is of no interest. It is a waste of time and energy and guarantees zero results. It is therefore necessary, before launching into demonstrations where one is ready to communicate one's experience with full intelligence and sincerely, to establish a preliminary diagnosis of the mental attitude of the person requesting information.

CHAPTER 4

SPECIAL TECHNIQUES TO IMPROVE THERAPY

*E*very country has developed its own approach to natural medicine, with specific orientations and special application techniques. In general, the final objective is the same: to find the best systems of defending and healing the body. The philosophy behind all types of natural medicine consistently place responsibility back on the individual–rather than the doctor–for the ultimate condition of his or her health. An unavoidable consequence of this individual (and family) responsibility is the need for more training and education in techniques for the repair and maintenance of the marvelous machines which have been entrusted to us for this life: our bodies.

Just as each country adds to the world's aromatic richness by contributing the best of its flora, so do naturopaths and other doctors from all over the world contribute to the expansion and improvement of natural medicine.

Through my international exposure I often see fascinating enhancements to practices and methods; practices and that deserve to be taken beyond the borders of their country of origin. With this first book my desire is to make known a few complementary techniques that are effective, relatively simple to put into practice, and do not require an unreasonable financial outlay.

If you buy top quality jogging shoes to run three times a year, it is just a waste of money! But if you jog regularly–three or four times a week–you will reap immense benefit from your investment and it will pay off handsomely. So it is with the equipment used in these techniques. It is for daily care, and although there is some expense involved, it is not unreasonable, and if these techniques become regular habits, the investment will be very worthwhile.

The first technique is an extremely effective method for cleansing the nasal cavities, combining refloxotherapy with a hydro-saline pulsated system developed by Hydro Floss®.

The second, a logical sequel to the above, is a special system of energized aerosoltherapy that is both silent and directional, called Osmobiosol®. This system was employed at home for the permanent nighttime care of Abby and also for that of a small Australian boy in Adelaide, treated for acute pneumonia.

The third technique involves the massage of the sinus and nasal zones, especially the mechanical unblocking of the internal orbital point, with a curved glass rod.

The fourth technique is the spirexotherapy method of massage, for use with floral waters..

These four techniques give the therapist and the patient remarkable new potential for respiratory and ENT therapy. A fifth technique, an extraction procedure for sucking out poisonous substances, is not directly connected with respiratory or ENT problems, but it is possible to extend its use to other high-risk accidental circumstances.

SECTION I

DAILY HYGIENE OF THE NASAL CAVITIES WITH THE HYDRO FLOSS®: A TECHNIQUE WITH POTENTIAL FOR PROFOUND RESULTS

The act of breathing is the first physiological function that allows us to live. In world-wide seminars and lectures I teach the slogan: "To breathe is to live and to breathe well is to live well!" The corollary is also true: to breathe poorly is to live poorly, both physiologically and psychologically.

This respiratory function takes place in all the cells of our body, on the biochemical and even on the electronic level. In reality, it is within the mitochondria of the cells that oxygen plays its part as the combustion agent that enables the burning up of fuels or nutrients coming from the digestive process.

Human beings breathe through the nose and not through the mouth, except in exceptional circumstances. Symbolically, the Bible talks about the "breath of life" as coming through the nose, not through the mouth. When we think of breathing as a physiological process, it is clear that air passing through the nose is more prepared to penetrate the lungs. It is warmed up, humidified and freed of numerous particles and microbes that are potentially damaging to the mucous membranes of the larynx, the trachea and the bronchi. When the nose is encumbered by too much mucous or is completely blocked, one has to breathe through the mouth, an abnormal situation.

Modern medicine can accomplish miracles in the realms of technology, surgery and reanimation, but when it comes to simple problems like a blocked nose, a cold or sinus problems, it has practically no satisfying solutions to offer. Vaso-constrictor medicines may give the illusion of cleared nostrils, but they can be an extremely dangerous trap, and I strongly recommend against using them. Their repeated use can lead to a state of dependence very difficult to overcome. I have known patients who used these products for years and could not quit, resulting in a desperate addiction.

Over a period of time, regular use of essential oils can greatly improve respiratory ventilation. But when a patient has serious problems with his nostrils, or feels frequently or even permanently stuffed up, or drips constantly (through the nose or back of the throat), immediate help is essential.

The Hindus, with their ancient Ayurvedic medicine, have been aware of the importance of assuring a free and easy air passage through the upper respiratory organs. Working with a respiratory discipline known as Pranayama, they know that each nostril corresponds to a subtle energetic trajectory inside the body.

Moreover, in experimental pathology, doctors have discovered a fact that is surprising to the Western scientific mind. They blocked one nostril in an experimental rabbit for a few weeks, then conducted a post-mortem on the animal. They noticed when examining the rabbit's lungs that the *lung on the side of the voluntarily blocked nostril had atrophied,* while the other one remained normal. By Western logic–a pure and simple mechanical logic–the air that comes in through the trachea should spread equally to both lungs, regardless of which nostril it goes through. This experiment showed that there must exist a supplementary circuit, probably of a subtle energetic nature, that connects each nostril to each lung.

In Ayurvedic practice, the nasal cavities are washed from a container with an outlet that is applied to the nostril opening. With the head leaning to one side the liquid flows through the nostril. The system is perfect...but only for human beings who are almost perfect themselves! A Yogi living in the mountains, breathing pure air, eating frugally, is not very likely to complain about a blocked-up nose. This technique for cleansing the nasal cavities amounts to an energy plus for an already very healthy person.

On the other hand, for the average Westerner who breathes polluted air, who eats excessively and too often eats the wrong kind of food, who is often forced to live a sedentary life, we know that the respiratory tracts are attacked by outside pollutants and mucosa from the digestive process. When a patient comes with a stuffed or completely plugged-up nose, the Ayurvedic nasal cleansing technique lacks in effectiveness or does not work at all. As I said earlier, it requires a context of existing purity, which is practically impossible for the average European, American, or Japanese. In these conditions, it is necessary to play a different card for efficiency, combining some kind of gentle mechanical action to provide greater stimulation and response.

The challenge with all of this has been to find an ideal instrument, one that would be effective and easy to use, to bring about a rapid cleansing. I thought I could use one of the popular oral irrigation systems or home-type atomizers available for the home care of gums and teeth. In France there are several easily available brands, and I purchased a model from each of the well-known brands, then tried them all to make a comparison. These systems are made for oral hygiene, but my goal was to use them in connection with the cleansing of the nasal cavities. I was not completely satisfied with any of them, but I had to be content with what was available.

At one particular training session in Paris on the therapeutic use of colors, I decided to explore a nearby store that specialized in imported health articles. Still preoccupied by the idea of finding a good technical solution to the cleansing of nasal cavities, I was attracted by a model I had never seen before. This was an appliance imported from the USA called the Hydro Floss®. I bought it and I tried it the same day in the hotel bathroom. I immediately realized, or rather my nose did–as a result of my longtime habit of pulsating hydrotherapy of the nasal cavities–that I finally had found what I had been seeking. It is as if I had been wearing, up to that point, shoes that were not made for my feet, so to speak, and on this fine day, I was putting my feet into a pair of shoes that were made exactly for them. We would say in French that they fit like a pair of gloves!

The Hydro Floss® is a very original piece of equipment because it magnetizes the solution for greater effectiveness in removing plaque. Very precise odonto-stomatological controlled studies have confirmed the superiority of the Hydro Floss® action to combat the problem of dental plaque. I will not elaborate further in this paragraph on this very technical aspect.

I only want to discuss its cleansing function, the cleansing of the nasal cavities, and on the results it brings. First, I will outline the specific advantages of the Hydro Floss® system.

1. The shape of the hydro jet, its impact, and its contact with the mucosa are particularly pleasant. The tip of the nozzle does not have a "douchette" setting, but nevertheless the penetration of the jet in the nasal cavities is very acceptable, we could say almost like a caress. It is definitely more comfortable to use than other systems.

2. The settings for the intensity of the jet are well calculated, ranging from a very low setting to a very strong one, which allows a very fine gradation according to the ability of the mucosa to withstand the pulsating massaging jet stream.

3. The systems commonly available do not allow separate adjustment of pulsation frequency or of jet propulsion intensity. This means that when we want to start with a low intensity, we must accept a very slow rhythm. Now this slowed rhythm is <u>not</u> ideal for nasal care (and the same is true for gums). The great advantage of Hydro Floss® technology over other oral irrigators I am familiar with is that it can hold the same pulsating rhythms whatever the jet's propulsive intensity may be. For the nasal cavities, we must start with a rather low intensity, and in all cases we never reach the maximum intensity, which would be too aggressive for the mucous membrane, which is more delicate than the gums. Consequently, unless we are using the Hydro Floss®, we will never experience the advantages of an appropriate rhythmic massage. We will see the importance of this rhythmic aspect on the level of reflexotherapy (the stimulation of the nervous endings).

4. The above advantages are complemented by another important asset, in the context of aromatherapeutic use, namely, the Hydro Floss®' ability to handle salinated aromatic solutions. In many oral irrigators, the propulsion circuit will not accept the solutions required for maximum and immediate therapy. The Hydro Floss® unit does not seem to have this problem, which is critical for our application.

Latent sinusitis: a wide-spread unresolved condition

My professional career in aromatic medicine lead me to a particular interest in the care of the respiratory organs, whether it be the bronco-pulmonary system or the realm of the ENT. Also, my teaching of theory, practice and technique has given me the opportunity to conduct tests on the sinus conditions of students and therapeutic practitioners attending my seminars. Whether in students or in patients, I have observed that sinus inflammation to some degree is a very common universal problem!

I am not talking about the acute frontal sinusitis causing sharp pains with evident signs of infections. I am talking about a permanent minor state of inflammation, or an apparently silent congestion of the mucosa, especially those of the frontal sinuses. The very simple test that will show the existence of this condition consists in applying a certain pressure, for example with the thumb, exactly on the inside of the orbit below the eye (See Photo No. 22). In most cases, even a moderate pressure triggers a wince, a pain and sometimes a scream. Either way, the person is surprised to notice to what extent the area is sensitive.

This sensitivity should not be considered normal just because many people experience it. We have too much of a tendency to mix up what is common or frequent with what is normal. Now, the norm expresses an idea of honesty and uprightness that can be understood in a physical, a moral, a physiological and psychological sense. Cancer, for example, has become, in our chemically-polluted world, quite a common occurrence. But still, it is not normal to die of cancer, even if it is quite logical to do so when we think of the aggressive actions of multiple factors engendered by the industrial world. The best proof that this sinusitis situation is not normal comes from the results obtained from regular aromatic care, especially from the use of a pulsating cleansing and purification of the nasal cavities with a saline hydro-aromatic solution. In fact, with time, the congestion of the mucosa declines, the nasal cavities become clearer, and the test of internal orbital pressure point shows little or no sensitivity.

The persistence of inflammation in the nasal cavities and the mucosa does not have merely local consequences. I have already pointed out, in the context of energetic circuits, the damaging effects of long-term obstruction to one of the nasal openings. The drippings of infected mucosa in the back of the pharynx, that then travel down toward the bronchi or that is swallowed to end up in the stomach, constitute a continuing aggressive attack on the body's defenses. We also know that infections of the middle ear (otitis) originate in the rhino-pharynx, then move on to attack the middle ear by way of the eustachian tube.

But there are still other consequences, which are deeper and more serious. We must remember that the turcic saddle that protects the pituitary gland is in a contiguous position with the upper nasal passages (ethmoidal sinus, sphenoidal sinus). A minimal but semi-permanent state of infection or inflammation brings with it irritation of the pituitary function. We are not talking about diseases per se, but rather minor irregularities, not serious enough to be considered pathological, but serious enough to have a negative effect on total glandular function. The endocrine system is comparable to an orchestra having as its conductor the pituitary-hypothalamus. We could say that the orchestra continues to play, but its harmony is broken by a certain number of wrong notes and by an uneven rhythm. This is all the more important for the fact that the anterior part of the pituitary has control of all the other glands (thyroid, adrenals, ovaries, or testicles).

Beyond the pituitary, we come in contact with the hypothalamic zone, which plays a major part in the regulation of basic behaviors. Another crucial aspect resides in the presence of a network of terminal nerves inside the nasal cavities. The soft and regular stimulation of these fibers provided by the salinated rhythmical hydro-aromatic massage proves to be a major asset for parasympathetic and sympathetic re-balance. This is obtained without any aggression and without trauma, through daily care provided at home.

As we work at the purification and cleansing of this zone, we trigger a complete process that influences positively, over time, the entire glandular-neuro system, and finally the psyche. Just as there are reflex zones in the bottom of the feet that we must liberate and activate by the massage, there are also endo-nasal reflexes for which the Hydro Floss® brings remarkable and complete care.

How to start nasal cleansing and purification

Pulsating hydro-aromatic nasal care is an authentic therapeutic procedure, and should be used regularly. If one decides to start this procedure and invest in the necessary equipment, it will not do to be enthused about it for a few days then put it aside or remember it occasionally. It is much simpler to make nasal purification a part of a regular, normal, and necessary personal hygiene, such as teeth and gum care. After brushing, when the teeth are cleaned, you just add to the routine one more step, a step that represents a higher level of care.

For teeth and gums one can use plain water without any problem. But for the nasal mucosa, I have observed that non-salinated water is a little bit irritating. Just as in a pharmacy we can find a physiological serum or diluted sea water to insert or atomize in the nostrils, we can prepare for ourselves (rather easily and cheaply) a reconstituted aqueous saline solution, that can also be made slightly aromatic with essential oils.

To do that, we first prepare the aromatic salt in a glass container with a tight lid. We put in it 8 tablespoons of fine sea salt. In France we have available sea salt from Guérance, which is rich in oligo-elements. (We also find salt flower which is the highest quality product available corresponding to the extra fraction of the Ylang Ylang essential oil). Each person will act according to his/her budget; but for the sake of health and vitality, investing in quality will certainly bring results worthy of a small sacrifice.

For this quantity of salt, 10 to 20 drops of essential oils should be added. The drops are mixed in one at a time with the handle of a wooden spoon or a wooden chopstick. The essential oil mixes well with fine salt. We can use either a single essential oil, for example the Melaleuca alternifolia, or a blend of oils, choosing always non-irritating essential oil varieties. The following is a simple and synergistic oil blend for this purpose:

3 ml   Melaleuca alternifolia

1 ml   Rosemary, verbenone or cineole

(We can test other mixtures and focus on the therapeutic side according to problems that may occur. For example, a young lady having problems with irregularity in her menstrual cycle may need to include a small quantity of essential oil from Clary Sage.)

Place this mixture of salt and essential oils in the bathroom and mix up only the needed amount each time you perform the procedure.

To begin the procedure, pour slightly warm water in a bowl or basin (hot water tends to congest the nasal mucosa) and add 1 to 2 teaspoons (2.5g to 5g) of the aromatic salt. Since we are not doing a vein injection but a nasal cleansing, we have a certain margin to play with and each person will judge what's right for him- or herself according to the comfort and the results obtained. Once the salt is in the water and mixed well, we just put the cannula/tube in the water and start the machine at highest intensity for 10 seconds (See Photo Nos. 17 and 18). Then we can begin the actual treatment.

With our head over the basin, the cannula is placed at the opening of one nostril and we turn on the appliance, starting at a low intensity.

Experience has shown that the more stuffiness or congestion there is, the more likely it is that some pain will be felt. (With the Hydro Floss®, which is a gentler machine than others, the pain will not be as great and it will be less frequent.) This reaction indicates that care is really needed; we just need to take it easy and go forward carefully as we progress toward complete recovery. As we persevere, the pain we may have felt at the beginning decreases and finally disappears, as a local improvement is felt along with a general feeling of well-being, freedom and purification (See Photo No. 19).

In the beginning, cleanse each nostril for 20 seconds. Then slowly increase the cleansing time to 1 minute per nostril. Make sure the jet goes in all directions to be sure the cleansing is complete and also to stimulate all the various reflex zones, like we would with a massage on reflex points of the feet. For faster and more profound results, this treatment should be performed morning and night.

All patients who have tried other systems and compared them to the Hydro Floss® quickly notice the difference and, like the introductory brochure says, fall in love with the new system. As for children, I begin having them do nasal cleansing, very gently, at age 4. Usually, the first treatment is done at the medical office and the patient, after 1 minute or so, is convinced of its benefit: Feeling this nasal liberation is like a revelation when one has suffered from congestion and inflammation for months or years, from a more or less permanent dripping, or from a more or less complete obstruction.

I frequently lend a machine to a patient to allow him to become aware of the positive effects.

Patients who are subject to allergic reactions will need to be prudent and use a lesser quantity of essential oils at first. By respecting the requirements of progress and observing well eventual reactions, these people also will derive genuine benefits from performing nasal cleansing. Once the nasal passages are free and clear, we can perform more refined complementary care. But this first step is indispensable to any other procedure.

The reader who learns this first step through this book and undertakes nasal cleansing seriously will be greatly rewarded for his or her efforts.

SECTION II

AEROSOLTHERAPY WITH THE OSMOBIOSOL®

In English-, and still more in German-speaking countries, the available aerosol systems are for diffusing aromas as a sort of recreational fragrancing rather than as a therapy. Here again we see two different styles: the soft approach intended to create a pleasant, relaxing atmosphere for daydreaming or as a stimulant, and the hard approach intended to create fine particles of aromatic substance for penetration through the respiratory interface. The appliances currently used in France function with an air spray from a glass container producing true aerosols, that is to say a propulsion of micro-particles of essential oils.

The Osmobiosol®–a system I have been perfecting for 20 years–is not for ambiance diffusion but rather for deep penetration through the respiratory interface. When I began working in medical aromatherapy, I was confronted with numerous diseases of the respiratory system and in the ENT sphere. This led me to develop several sophisticated respiratory care systems for medical office use, available only to professionals because of the considerable financial investment involved.

At the same time I began exploring ways to make a device affordable enough and effective enough for regular home health care. The glass containers used on the original systems had wide openings that made them noisy–a problem when used at night, especially when used with children. My first step, therefore, was to concentrate air flow, by narrowing the diameter of the output tubes. The second improvement was the development of a device for breaking down the particles to obtain a finer spray.

Realizing how difficult it was to keep active young children in front of ordinary aerosol devices, I focused on developing a system that would take advantage of the nighttime hours and help patients sleep more peacefully. With this approach, every hour spent breathing during sleep could be made beneficial for the respiratory tracts. A typical appliance sends particles upwards to diffuse throughout the room; it is not designed for focused individual care. I developed a way to output a fine essential oil mist through a narrow spray that could be directed toward a specific location. In treatment this enables us to concentrate the flow of aromatic molecules toward a patient's face and nostrils (See Photo No. 20).

In the final version, a spiral intermediary part was placed between the glass container and extension tube. All in all, the aerosol session takes place in a perfectly relaxed atmosphere, either at the medical office or at home, in an easy chair or in bed. In Abby's case, the system was operated every night above her face, to allow respiration of the essential oil particles during the "lost hours" of the night (See Photo No. 21). I keep several of these systems in my possession to loan to my patients when they need immediate intensive care. Parents immediately see the remarkable effectiveness of Osmobiosol® when used for their children, and they often purchase the device for themselves to help them take better control of their family's health.

Only the very best quality essential oils can be used in intensive or frequent use with the Osmobiosol®. The oils used must also be very mild in order not to create irritation of the mucous membrane. The oils must have no additive of any sort, whether alcohol, vegetable oil, DPG, etc. The essential oils of *Melaleuca alternifolia* or *Ravensara aromatica*, for example, are very successful. Since only small quantities are used at a time, more expensive oils can be considered, such as Green myrtle (of French origin)[31], especially for limited sessions.

In this general introduction of the Osmobiosol®, I do not want to enter into complex technical details. My intention is to bring the existence of this high performance system to the notice of medical or clinical therapists. Aerosoltherapy deserves theoretical and practical training at many levels, but that is not the object of this book.

The prerequisite for the success of aerosoltherapy is the release of the mucus blocking the nasal channels. This is why a logical two-step progression should be considered: begin with the Hydro Floss® and follow up with the Osmobiosol®. For nocturnal care it is preferable to have a regulator to start and stop the operation at regular intervals. The Osmobiosol® also makes it possible to carry out psycho-olfactory and ventilation work in depth, affecting both the body and the mind. These exciting aspects will be further developed in future publications.

The Osmobiosol® can also be used to propel very fine essential oil particles to destinations other than the nostrils: to the pharynx for example, or into tooth caries or the tympanum in the case of middle ear infection. It is advisable to be able to adjust the air flow, especially for local application.

Also, after an ESA aromatic massage treatment, it is advisable to leave the patient calm and relaxed for a while. An Osmobiosol® treatment pleasantly ends, prolongs and completes an aromatic massage session.

The following striking phenomenon took place with this highly beautiful olfactory essential oil:

> A female patient came to me for an exam and after taking her blood pressure, the figures were alarming–around 240/150! I decided to put her under the Osmobiosol® using only this essential oil, diffused above her face, close to the nostrils. After 20 minutes, her blood pressure had returned almost to normal! This illustrates the importance of the neuro-vegetative receptors in the nasal cavity. These receptors receive the fine aromatic particles, their effect being reinforced with the highly sedative olfactory influence of the green myrtle essential oil. Furthermore, with this form of aromatic treatment the particles really penetrate into the bloodstream via the pulmonary pathway. The treatment is thus complete in itself, bringing together the Matter, Energy and Information from "Dr Pénoël's Aromatic Triad." During introductory courses I taught in England for the intensive application of essential oils, the inhalation of green myrtle essential oil with the Osmobiosol® was found to be a profoundly relaxing experience, for body and soul!

SECTION III

SPIREXOTHERAPY, A COMPLETE HEALTH MAINTENANCE METHOD FOR PROFESSIONALS AND FOR THE FAMILY

As in the case of the Osmobiosol®, I have been working for the last 20 years on a very special and high performance system known as spirexotherapy. I can already see the question on your lips: "Now then, Doctor Pénoël, you're not going to tell us there is a high performance method not already known outside of France?" My answer is "Yes, there is," and I am going to give you a couple of examples of the difficulty of spreading good techniques across national borders and even within one's own country.

The first example concerns the irrigation of the colon, which is a classical method in naturopathy and has been practiced for decades, especially in the U.S. I personally discovered this technique at the office of a naturopathic practitioner while in Australia (on a visit to Perth after cross-ing the 2,500 Km of the Nullarbor Plain). On returning to France, we attended a training course in London, England, in order to apply this method. I was surely one of the first French doctors to practice hydro-therapy of the colon, back in 1988; The technique has now become wide-spread in France, but we had to wait a decade! In this example, the transfer went from the U.S. to France. When the transfer goes in the opposite direction, from France to the U.S., it takes even longer and is more difficult.

The second demonstration concerns a health method known as Natural Hygiene, which exists at the nutritional level, of the dissociation of certain food categories regarded as incompatible with the digestive system. The late Dr. H.M. Shelton, who worked in a dieting and natural care center in San Antonio, Texas, was one of the pillars of this method. You would think this method would have become widespread decades ago. Not at all. For years it was only practiced confidentially in countries with large popula-tions like the U.S. What happened? It needed a dynamic young couple, thoroughly convinced of its benefits, to get hold of the method and dedicate their lives to spreading it not only in North America but over most parts of the world. Fit for Life by Harvey and Marilyn Diamond (Warner Books 1985) rapidly became a bestseller in English and subsequently internationally.

I am certain the moment has come for spirexotherapy to pass the French frontier and be introduced to the rest of the world, beginning with the U.S.

A Bit of History

Every invention begins with someone's idea. For spirexotherapy we have to go back to the 1950s in France. In the years immediately after World War II, my country was recovering from war and enemy occupation and the economy was not exactly flourishing. The family laundry, for example, was done by hand, and in order to clean dirty linen more effectively, a bright Frenchman, Roland Degré, got the idea of making a device to exert a combined pressure/suction on the material. He brought out a prototype and was satisfied with the results. That was the first historic step. But the story did not stop there.

One day, a physiotherapist discovered the appliance. Knowing the human body well, he saw at once the highly valuable application which could result from its use on the body. He therefore began working on the first model for physiotherapy purposes and did in fact obtain very positive results, confirming his initial intuition. After all, the human tissue also needs to be cleansed of congesting toxins and freed from the accumulated refuse which impedes its functioning.

From this beginning, additional models were perfected and introduced. But the basic principles remained the same, since the functioning of the human body has also remained the same ever since man has been on the earth.

The Principles Behind Spirexotherapy

First of all, we need to answer a question. Do you know where the vital interchanges take place, those which allow oxygen to spread through the tissues and cells and carbon dioxide to fill the lungs? You realize, I am sure, the crucial importance of this nutrient/energy exchange at the foundation of life. I explained in the section on the Hydro Floss® that true breathing takes place inside the cell (in the mitochondria). But for this internal combustion to take effect, the supply of oxygen and proper evacuation of residues, particularly carbon dioxide, must be assured. It is not enough to breathe in and out correctly. Surely, good pulmonary ventilation is the very first step (and if possible with clean air!), just as a blower fans the fire in the hearth. But if the wood is packed too tightly there is little chance of the blower doing its job properly, however hard it blows. The air blown on to the flame must circulate freely and actively. If the kindling, branches, and logs are placed in a more open fashion, the air will circulate quickly, bringing indispensable oxygen for proper combustion. The flame will mount, radiant with warmth and light!

For life to shine with radiance in our bodies it is just the same. What is the answer to our question? Yes, it is the blood circulation system. But let us go further with the examination of this vital system. It all starts at the heart and returns to the heart, through a major circulation system (the whole body) and a minor circulation system (the lungs). First, the large, medium and small arteries, then the large, medium and small arterioles carry the blood to the farthest and most intimate zones. But the most fantastic network in the body is that of the capillary vessels. It is here we find the ultimate answer to our question: the interchange takes place at the capillaries, which are even finer than hair. Have you any idea of the length of the capillary network in one human body? It has been estimated at 100,000 Km, two and a half times the circumference of the earth! Not only do gaseous exchanges take place at this level (red blood cells), but also the functions of immune-defense and counter attack (white blood cells). Stagnation, slow-down, congestion, blockage, are synonymous with weakness, toxicity, loss of vitality, lessening of the faculty of defense, and counter-attack. There exist few ways of specifically activating capillary circulation. Conventional electric vibrators do not have the capillary acti-vating capacity necessary for meaningful improvement.

In order to create a powerful and specific effect, the spirex has a series of small suction pads, which are applied to the skin surface. These suction pads immediately bring to mind those the octopus uses to trap its prey. The important difference being the rotating movement, which makes it possible to shift the pads. For maximum suction it is important to work on damp ground. Some therapeutic action can also be obtained by working dry, but it is not as effective because the suction or aspiratory phase, which plays a primary role, is greatly reduced. I therefore recommend coupling the use of the spirex with floral water or diluted essential oils for maximum results. When the spirex is used on moistened skin, a radiant pinkness of the skin very soon appears on the treated zone. This pinkness is very different from the redness caused by irritation (as might be produced by a friction glove). It shows simply, visibly, that capillary circulation is being activated, *which is the primary therapeutic function of spirexotherapy* (See Photo No. 24).

As a complement to the suction effect there is an effect of rhythmic percussion, which automatically occurs as the spirex passes over the surface of the skin. We thus have the means to create simultaneous rhyth-mic percussion and aspiration in a way that is easy to use and exception-ally effective. Spirexotherapy is a holistic method, providing local, regional, and general systemic action on all parts of the body.

The Effectiveness of Spirexotherapy Demonstrated
by Practical Examples

There exist several spirexotherapy appliances, but the two principal ones are supra-spirex and facial spirex. For sensitive, fragile, traumatized zones it is preferable to use the facial spirex, which is very easy to handle and can be used with very low pressure. The supra-spirex is more voluminous and exerts stronger suction/pressure. It is more suitable for working large, solid areas, particularly along the spinal column (See Photo No. 27).

Spirexotherapy occupies a special place in the practice of the Osmobiotic® method. Spirexotherapy works well for treating a particular problem and for giving stimulating therapy for general fitness and well-being. In the latter case, which has an energizing aim, the spirexotherapy is coupled with ESA aromatherapy using diluted essential oils in regular sessions. Typically, this would involve a series of four to six complete sessions, at a rate of one or two sessions per week. Training in spirexotherapy should be a practical course. The student must first of all thoroughly understand the underlying theory; after this preliminary phase he should:

- watch a treatment
- receive a treatment
- treat another person
- learn how to use the spirex on himself.

These four complementary stages will allow him to acquire a solid basis for working in good conditions.

Here is an example of a general treatment. It took place in April 1992 on the occasion of the publication of the first edition of this book in French.

In Paris, during the Soft Medicine Exhibition, my wife and I gave a lecture on aromatherapy followed by a practical workshop during which spirexotherapy was demonstrated. One of the people present, a woman in her 50s, complained of a semi-permanent state of nervous tension she had been suffering from for years. The inability to relax, to "switch off," is due to a number of causes, chiefly psychological, whether conscious or unconscious. During a public demonstration of spirexotherapy it was, of course, impossible to psychoanalyze the lady in question. She was given her spirexotherapy treatment, especially along the spinal column. The manual rhythmic vibration with suction/percussion, accompanied by a diluted extract of real lavender, very quickly (in the course of 10 minutes) produced such a deep release that she fell asleep for a while on the demonstration table!

It may seem obvious, but I will mention it for the record: The spirex does not replace normal hand work, and the bare hand can never accomplish the same work as the spirex. Both are complementary, the hand work following logically after the application of the spirex.

Here is an another example of spirexotherapy, this time with the facial spirex in an extreme case. The following event illustrates the capacity of the spirex to resolve even the most delicate situations:

It concerns a German lady who took part in a course organized in the Drôme. She had suffered a serious leg accident and had undergone several surgical operations (grafts), which had left her with an extreme sensitivity at the traumatized and operated zone. She suffered sharp local pain at the slightest touch, and nothing had succeeded in improving this difficult situation. Even very gentle manual aromatic ointments had brought no improvement. During my lecture to Swiss and German aromatherapists, my wife suggested an aroma spirexotherapeutic treatment, which she accepted. Using the supra-spirex was out of the question, because its effect was much too strong for a hypersensitive zone. Rose-Marie started very gently along the edge of the painful zone. A cloth was impregnated with a diluted aromatic solution and was used to cover the leg. The secret of the spirex is in this very special rhythmic percussion movement which, little by little, anesthetized, put to sleep, relaxed and soothed the area which had been giving her trouble for 12 years. The pressure was increased gradually until the hypersensitivity began to decline. This required infinite patience with a patient who had suffered for so many years and who physically and psychologically was in great fear as the hypersensitive zone was touched. Patience and gentleness were rewarded with good results. My wife spent more than an hour applying the facial spirex with aromatic extracts. At the end of the session the patient was able to accept manual massage of the traumatized zone for the first time in 12 years. She of course immediately bought a facial spirex in order to continue the treatment at home.

I want to return now to the treatment to be given in the case of local trauma. We have already talked about using essential oil of peppermint to relieve pain in such a case. Doing this immediately can soothe intense pain and this is highly important. But it is not enough. Especially in the case of an impact near the tibia, the periosteum is very close induration zones form which do not disappear by themselves. I recommend the use of the facial spirex to dissolve these hardened zones. If we allow them to persist, these zones create blockages along the body's energetic pathways, which can have serious repercussions, whose origins are all but impossible to determine.

Let me tell you an anecdote. Tomato plants are transplanted in France during the month of May. When I was doing this I knocked the supports into the ground with a wooden stick. I missed a stroke and the stick hit my right tibia, on the inside just above the ankle. It was very painful and I immediately put a few drops of essential oil of peppermint on the spot. As always, the anesthetizing effect took place rapidly and I was able to continue working . I took no other care, which was a mistake on my part. In any case, two weeks after the incident, when I felt no spontaneous pain, I touched the traumatized spot. What a surprise! I realized there remained a terribly sensitive spot, in fact an extremely painful one, even at the slightest touch, whereas I felt nothing in the absence of contact...Peppermint essential oil is indispensable, but it is not sufficient for what in medicine is termed a "resolvent," that is to say, able to dissolve the micro-calcifications and micro-crystals that form at the place of impact.

This allowed me to test, in my own flesh, the effectiveness of the facial spirex. I prepared a diluted aromatic solution (true lavender, geranium, verbenone rosemary) to soak a compress for putting round the bottom of my leg. I began to work with the facial spirex, very gently at first and on the edge of the hypersensitive area, then approaching this zone and little by little increasing the pressure (See Photo Nos. 25 and 30). You have to give yourself time for this sort of care. I had three 20 minute sessions in all during the day. At the end of the day I could feel definite improvement; it was still sensitive, due in part to the intensive spirexation. But, the next day it was possible to massage the previously hypersensitive zone by hand without causing intense pain.

In one case, which caused me great surprise, a pain and blockage that had lasted for a year disappeared after 5 minutes treatment with the spirex. The patient was a businessman in his 50s, a grandfather who had fallen when playing ball with his grandson. For 12 months he complained of a residual pain in the wrist that had cushioned the fall. No ointment had succeeded in soothing the pain. He was passing through the Drôme at the time and took the opportunity of visiting with me. I suggested a very simple treatment, namely the application of the supra-spirex. After 5 minutes treatment on his wrist, he could move it freely without feeling any more pain. I know such cases appear to be invented, but it is the strict truth. Examples of spectacular and relatively rapid effects obtained with spirexotherapy are frequent in the medical field and in daily life.

Other Examples of Treatment

For the local treatment of sinusitis we use the facial spirex, passing it in an up and down movement above the frontal and maxillary sinuses, as well as over the nasal bone and the sides of the nose. For a sore throat and tonsillitis, we pass the spirex along the side of the neck (See Photo Nos. 28). In both cases it is necessary to gently unblock the nape of the neck, therefore to pass the spirex from the occipital bone to the trapezius. If the diluted aromatic liquid cannot always be applied, the effect of passing the spirex over a shirt brings about a release of the tension which occurs in all ENT infections.

Spirexotherapy is shown to be very useful in the treatment of the abdomen, especially for activating the intestines and untying the solar plexus, which is often knotted in people suffering from stress.

Spirexotherapy is a powerful means for preparing athletes for action and above all for acquiring proper relaxation after their effort. If we take the example of prolonged jogging, as for a 10K or even a marathon, the calves are sure to need special care to free the accumulated tensions and micro-traumas. The jogger lies on his front on the treatment table, with this feet over the edge. The person giving the treatment uses his thigh to exert a slight pressure on the balls of the feet in order to stretch the gastrocnemius muscles. The aromatic solution is spread over the calves and treatment is applied with the supra-spirex (See Photo No. 29). The jogger will rapidly feel great relief. The calves are treated, followed by the thighs. The patient then turns over and the spirex is passed over the front of the legs and thighs. The spirex treatment may be prolonged with an ordinary manual aromatic massage. But there is no comparison for the rapid action and deep release and the intense draining of toxins obtained with the spirex.

For treatment of the thorax, spirexing is done along the sternum and ribs. The spirex can be employed in any direction, but it is important to follow a parallel trajectory obliquely across the ribs. The arms, forearms, wrists, and hands also derive great benefit from spirexotherapy, which is perfectly understandable when one considers the important Chinese meridians which run through the upper members of the body.

There is one contra-indication to the employment of spirexotherapy which must be mentioned. This is gout. The problem is linked to the uric acid deposit in the joints and special treatment against uric acid is needed.

Spirexotherapy produces a favorable action on the circulation in the lower members of the body, especially for people who have to work standing up for long periods. A young dental assistant in her 20s came to consult me about circulation problems she was having due to standing virtually immobile beside the dentist's chair. She loved her job, but had to find an effective solution to help offset the consequences of this stagnation. She had found initial relief in taking plant extracts orally and in local massage. After I recommended the spirex every evening after work she experienced remarkable improvement and was able to carry on with the work she loved.

Where a patient has large varicose veins the spirex should not be passed across the swollen veins, but it can be passed around them. In such sensitive cases it is better to work with the facial spirex, which is gentler and easier to handle. Based my experience, spirexotherapy is a method applicable both by health professionals and by the family at home.

It was not my intention in this section to provide full training on the subject, but to provide a simple introduction. Spirexotherapy, like other techniques described in this chapter, must be experienced to be fully appreciated. When I give a demonstration on a person chosen among those present at a seminar, and they experience first-hand the incredible relaxing effects of working on the back and spinal column, the value of the spirex becomes very clear.

SECTION IV

PERI-ORBITAL AND NASAL MASSAGE
WITH THE CURVED GLASS ROD

Appliances such as the Hydro Floss®, the Osmobiosol®, and Spirexotherapy instruments, represent an investment that, though not unreasonable, requires reflection. In particular you need to know yourself and decide whether you are prepared to take a serious step and follow it through. I talk of "Aromatic Discipline" for a very good reason: There must be some sense of commitment and personal discipline before we encourage a patient to acquire home techniques that enable him/her to become more and more independent and responsible. Only about 3 percent of the average population is able to submit to a regular and conscientious discipline. (For people already involved in the daily use of essential oils this proportion perhaps increases tenfold!) In any case, the aid proposed in this section is very simple to use and produces an excellent result at a reasonable cost.

In this section I will return to the "ouch point," the highly sensitive point at the internal angle of the orbit, detected in almost all who have never undertaken a cleansing, purifying, and unblocking process of the sinus and nasal zones. Massage on this point is highly important, supplementing the Hydro Floss® and Osmobiosol® treatments. It can be done with the cushion of the thumb or the index finger. The finger cushion by definition, however, consists of flesh that greatly reduces the pressure, unless intensely applied, which is not easy to do for a massage that has to last for some minutes! I therefore recommend the use of a glass rod with a curved end, which provides precise and intense pressure without a great deal of effort (See Photo No. 23).

I must give a warning about the direction of the massage application. In facial esthetic treatment, the beauty therapist normally follows the direction of the eyebrows, working outwards from the inside. From our point of view of draining the sinus cavities, do you think this is the correct direction? Not according to the evidence. The secretions have to be brought *toward* the nostrils, so that they can be eliminated. We do not want to turn it away from its natural exit. When we compare this with the direction of abdominal massage, we observe that it must be done clockwise—and not counter-clockwise—to ease the intestinal passage outwards from the body. The massage direction, depending on the zone and the purpose of the massage, is of great importance. Massage of the lower edge of the sub-orbital zone, of the floor of the frontal sinus, proceeding outwards, could provoke a sinusal crisis, that is, reawaken the latent sinusitis previously described.

In practice, the release of the most sensitive spot, at the upper internal angle of the eye, should be done progressively and gently. This zone, already very sensitive to manual pressure, should not be attacked at the same pressure with the glass rod. Apply the curved end of the rod to the lower orbital face, *starting at the outside and working inward toward the very sensitive point above the internal angle of the eye.* After ten movements or so, concentrate on the most sensitive point, continuing the movement inward. The pressure can be increased progressively, but it is better not to rush matters for the first few days. The upper infra-orbital massage is completed by massaging, in the same direction, the edge of the lower orbit. Massage is concentrated after that on the nose itself, primarily at the top, moving downward, followed by the wings, all with an inward movement.

Like the hands and feet, the face as a whole (the nose in particular) numerous reflex points. Treatment of the sinus is therefore completed by massage of the facial reflex zones. The glass rod can be applied dry, or with a drop of aromatized oil, provided concentration is very low (due to the nearness of the eye). For 5 ml of vegetable or calendula oil, add one drop of a mild essential oil such as rosemary, verbenone or cineole.

Sinus care with the glass rod can be done while pursuing other activities, such as watching the television, traveling by car, in an airplane, on the subway, or by train. The glass rod can, of course, be used on other parts of the body, especially on reflex points of the feet and toes. During an attack of sinusitis I have often eased the unblocking process by applying a vibratory complement to the inner angle of the eye. Professional methods of natural treatment of sinusitis, whether chronic or as an isolated eruption, will be dealt with in detail in future publications in this collection.

SECTION V

USING THE ASPIVENIN® OR EXTRACTOR® IN
INITIAL EMERGENCY TREATMENT

Whereas spirexotherapy remains confined to France, the Aspivenin has a well-deserved international reputation as a tool for extracting snake venom after a bite. I had the honor of getting to know Mr. André Emerit, the French engineer who invented this unique device, when he presented the prototype at the Inventors' Exhibition (for the Lépine Competition at the Paris Fair). Some young American students who were finishing their commercial studies had the good fortune to discover the system and they decided to make it known in North America, where the name was changed to "The Extractor." Having emigrated to Australia three years after knowing about the Extractor®, I tried to introduce the system there in 1985, but I met with considerable resistance. Since Australian snakes have very different fangs from their cousins in the Northern Hemisphere, there was a complete barrier on the part of the Australian authorities. What I want to show here is that there are many possibilities for the use of the Extractor®, other than the field of herpetology.

I must first of all make it clear that we are here in the same situation as the Hydro Floss®. We are using these devices for purposes quite different than their inventors had originally conceived. My purpose is to provide information, knowing that others, whether or not members of the medical profession, will be able to benefit themselves, their families, or their patients. We saw that the spirex was born from the idea of washing laundry and its end use is quite different. In the case of the Extractor® it is obvious that its initial function is still valid. It is quite simply a small suction pad linked to a sort of syringe, creating a vacuum for extracting poison injected by stings or bites.

The genius in Mr. Emerit's discovery was that he found a way to create a vacuum, not by pulling a piston, but by pushing it. The Extractor® can be operated with one hand–impossible with an ordinary syringe or plunger. The first time I used the Extractor® in an emergency was during a summer vacation three months after my discovery of it. Our son, then age 5, was paddling in the sea and he put his foot on the prickly spine on the back of a weever, a poisonous fish well known in the Mediterranean. He felt a searing pain under his toe. Fortunately we had the Extractor® with us and the poison was quickly extracted, bringing rapid relief.

The complementary use of the Extractor® in the world of therapy is for the extraction of infecting particles, especially where a wound is caused by a pointed article. I shall summarize the situation I personally experienced on two occasions (the event is described in detail in the first volume of the collection "Emergencies and Intensive Care," published in French). Both times the scenario was the same: On climbing into a dark loft I put my foot on a rusty nail coming up through a plank of wood. I gave a shout and lifted my foot with the plank attached to the nail buried in my flesh (See Photo No. 31). Immediate emergency care was called for. In this zone, the penetration of infecting particles constitutes an obvious danger. The advice I offer in no way prevents the subsequent intervention of health professionals. It was a case of first aid, as one may give in any number of accidents or unexpected health problems while waiting for a doctor or paramedic. We learn mouth to mouth resuscitation and CPR to try to save someone's life. But we implement these techniques while waiting for the paramedics, not as a substitute for them. But if these emergency efforts are not carried out at once, the chances of saving a patient can be greatly reduced.

The difference in my two adventures with the rusty nail was that I did not have the Extractor® in the first case, but I did have it in the second.. Without the Extractor®, however hard one tries to force out the blood by pressing the edges of the very small hole made by the point of the nail, evacuation is practically impossible at this part of the body. One even has the impression that the pressure pushes the potential infection further in. An external disinfectant, whether essential oil of *Melaleuca alternifolia* or the usual pharmaceutical products, does not extract the infecting particles carried deeply in by the nail. This happened on the first misadventure. I had to resort to drastic means (still in the field of natural medicine, but with sophisticated techniques I have in my care center).[26]

The second time, I immediately used the Extractor®, which at once brought out the blood about to be infected. I then applied intensive aromatic care, with essential oil of *Melaleuca alternifolia*, locally and along the leg and thigh, as far as the groin glands. There was no infection and I can confirm that the use of the Extractor® was largely responsible for a much faster healing cycle. I therefore advise my readers to include an Extractor® in their emergency kit (See Photo No. 32). I would not wish such accidents on anybody, but the possession of the Extractor® is rather like an insurance premium: we would rather not have to use it, but when an accident occurs we are happy to have thought of it.

Another case in which I strongly recommend using the Extractor is for wounds or pricks from fish bones or bone fragments (amongst butchery personnel hand or finger wounds from pork bones automatically cause infection). In any case, doctors, nurses, and naturopaths should have the Extractor® in their first aid kit and advise families to do the same.

We have now covered the important techniques one should know for the efficacy of aromatic care. There will be many other means which will be introduced and developed in the course of future publications. But for a first contact, this represents an important and complete program to be set up in progressive stages. This first book does not pretend to cover all the fields. Even a lifetime would not suffice…. In the context of Abby's adventure and that of the history of the Franco-Australian connection and subsequently with other English-speaking countries, I have chosen to develop certain priority themes, and bring a bit of light to bear in several fields. The "Integrated Aromatic Medicine" collection will continue, progressively and in detail, the theoretical, practical, and technical teaching in aromatic substances in the vast field of an open and wider medicine, which I call integrated, integrating, integral, and honest.

In this complete and responsible medical approach, priority is systematically given to the nutritional aspect. For this reason, in the next chapter Rose-Marie provides a number of simple recommendations and explains the recipes suggested for Abby's change of diet to give every chance of success in the intensive struggle undertaken in April 1986. As a complement to this nutritional advice, I have added some simple techniques for massaging the reflex points of the soles of the feet, and basic advice for learning to breathe better.

Footnotes:
26. Although a detailed description of these natural care techniques lies outside the scope of this first book, health professionals can find more detail in *Urgences et Soins Intensifs* due to appear later in English.

CHAPTER 5

FOOD, FEET, AND BREATH
with Rose-Marie Pénoël

INTRODUCTION

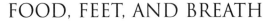

There is a saying in French which states:
Behind every success of a man, there is a major role played by a woman

ose-Marie has played this role during all our aromatic and life adventures. Having received real psychic gifts from her family (from her great grandmother who was already a healer), she has specialized not in trying to divine winning numbers to win the Lotto jackpot, but in helping all those who come to her to regain their physical and moral health and well-being. And, you will agree that, no matter how big a sum is won at the Lotto, if the winner loses his or her physical, emotional, mental and spiritual health, it becomes meaningless. (Of course maybe not for his or her heirs...)

From the introduction of this book with Abby's story, we have repeatedly stated that essential oils and aromatherapy, especially in the context of mucous accumulation in the respiratory system, can only exert their full restorative power when some dietary reform is accepted by the patient and the family.

Eating junk food everyday at a fast-food restaurant and hoping to improve one's health in a meaningful and long-lasting way, seem like nonsense, yet many think this way. The. knowledge and know-how that Rose-Marie will share with you is based on many thousands of experiences all over the world. You understand that Abby's case was chosen as a prototype, a symbolic example but the functioning of the respiratory system is the same in Los Angeles, in London, in Paris, in Oslo, in Athens, in Tel Aviv, as it is in Auckland or in Adelaide. In the next book (already available in French), I will explain in minute detail the physiological and pathological connections between the small intestine, the large intestine, the liver and the mucous membranes of the respiratory system. For this very first book, we will focus directly on the practical side of the nutritional approach, with simple, basic, healthy and tasty recipes.

The practical presentation of the food aspect in health maintenance will be complemented by the presentation of the foot aspect, i.e. reflexology as we have developed it in our clinic. We have decided to describe for the first time in a book a very special point that we call the "psy" point (psy = linked with psychological problems), discovered by Rose-Marie under providential inspiration. And to close this last chapter, RoseMarie will give some advice about simple breathing exercises.

INITIAL RECOMMENDATIONS FOR HEALTHY
AND FLAVORSOME NUTRITION

When it came to taking little Abby in hand, we had to support the aromatic medicine with sound nutrition.

I have often seen aromatherapy act in a spectacular way, especially at the start, but it then sometimes reaches a certain limit. One has the impression the treatment hits some kind of plateau. If at that moment, some simple corrective nutritional steps are accepted and applied by the patient and the patient's family, the doors open again as if by magic and the effects of the aromatic extracts are multiplied.

As we had to obtain a significant positive result in a very short time for Abby, there was no question that we would have to start nutritional care immediately with the aromatic treatment. We had to give the life force every possible chance.

The added difficulty in Abby's case was that her mother had already consulted nutritionists and believed she "knew it all." She did in fact have some interesting ideas, especially concerning the harmful influence of dairy foods on the production of mucus. But Sue made a number of mistakes, which had to be highlighted and corrected. When she at last humbly recognized that she still had things to learn, everything became possible.

The following had to be rectified from the very start:
- the daily consumption of peanut butter and "vegemite"
- the consumption of mucous-forming cereals
- morning orange juice
- and a few other errors, which taken together made a big influence

Orange juice, much too acidifying for such a thin and sickly child, was replaced by carrot juice, freshly extracted from organic carrots (not bottled). The corn, oats and rice regularly consumed by Abby as cereals in various forms were replaced by barley (flakes, cream, flour, pearl barley), millet (cream, flakes and seed) and potatoes.

Instead of peanut butter and "vegemite" I substituted flavorsome recipes based on tofu. As for eggs, only the yolks were used, the whites also being a source of sticky mucus (try using egg whites to make glue!).

The most important thing was to get the child to accept and like this new form of food, because she had become quite temperamental and demanding: already eating very little, she knew very well it was difficult to force or to refuse her.

Our nutritional advice thus became natural culinary art, harmonizing flavors to provide nourishment and give pleasure. This is an essential aspect of my approach: how often have I come across followers of natural food who are unable to make up balanced dishes that are both nourishing and satisfying to taste.

In this first publication, I shall limit myself by giving the basic recipes which encouraged little Abby to accept and follow a new way of eating, without frustration or lack of balance.

**To convert grams to ounces in the following recipes,
multiply the number of grams by .035.**

Natural sugar substitute

Industrial sugar, white or brown, has no place in my kitchen. From time to time I use cane sugar (pure sugar cane juice, simply dehydrated) or honey for sweetening herb teas. How do I replace sugar? Quite simply by using the fruit Nature provides, in the form of dried fruit. Here are my recipes for uncooked raisin jam, date jam and raisin/date jam.

For raisin jam: use 250 g of seedless organic raisins (sultanas) of a deep brown color. Rinse them and let them soak 5-6 minutes in very hot water. Drain, throw away the water, and put them in the mixer (without water). Finely grate the yellow and white rind of an organic lemon peel (but without the juice). Mix this to a thick puree.

For date jam: follow the same process with dates, after removing all the pits.

For the mixed raisin/date jam: mix together 200 g of raisin jam and 200 g of date jam.

Put this mixture in a closed receptacle in the refrigerator or storeroom (the lemon peel acts as a natural preservative).

The jams can be put in a pot for going on a journey and used for breakfast or snacks: spread on whole Melba toast. This natural jam is healthy and is loved by children young and old. Prepared in this way, it will serve for other sugared recipes.

Recipe for light pancakes (without milk) for 4 to 5 people
INGREDIENTS:

> Three cups or 300 g of cream of barley.
> One cup or 40 g of buckwheat flour.
> Four egg yolks, separated from the whites.
> Four and a half cups of water.
> Grated organic lemon peel (both the rind and the white);
> Two level tablespoons of raisin, date, or raisin/date jam.
> Soak a small pad of kitchen paper in a teaspoonful of unrefined oil (sunflower, carthamum, etc) and wipe the pan with this; the moistened pad will serve for all the pancakes. Heat the pan well, before putting in the batter for the first pancake.

PREPARATION OF THE BATTER:

> Break the eggs, throw away the whites and put the yolks in a bowl. Whisk, add the flour then the water little by little, stirring all the time, to obtain a smooth batter. Add the lemon rind and the jam; brush the pan with the oiled pad, and heat. Pour the mixture into the pan with a small ladle; brown each side (do not forget to cover with a perforated lid). After each pancake take the precaution of wiping the pan with the

pad (oiled once only, at the beginning). Place the pancakes in a dish. If they are not sweet enough, add more jam. Good eating!

You can follow the same procedure for savory pancakes. The proportions are the same, but the jam is replaced by different dried or fresh herbs (a tablespoon) and three pinches of salt. Grate carrots, zucchinis, and onions finely; slice some mushrooms. Oil the pan and fry the vegetables over a low heat. When cooked, add them to the batter. The vegetables can also be used to fill the pancakes. For those who cannot digest eggs, prepare the same recipes without egg yolks (or the whites, of course). This batter can be used for making sweet or savory pancakes.

IMPORTANT

For all recipes containing tofu, the tofu needs to be steamed for five minutes (place it in a strainer above boiling water, and cover); this reduces the purins. For recipes requiring cold tofu, simply allow it to cool after being steamed.

Recipe for savory tofu for 2 to 4 people (depending on the type of meal)

(This basic recipe eliminated the "vegemite" and peanut butter for Abby.)

Take 250 g of natural rinsed tofu (white block), an onion, a clove of garlic, a slice of sweet red pepper, a branch of parsley, a pinch of herbs, a tablespoon of cold-pressed unrefined oil, six black olives (washed and pitted), the juice of a small lemon, two capfuls of gastronomic Pianto or tamari. Put these ingredients in the mixer. When you get a smooth cream the recipe is ready. Above all, it must not be cooked. This preparation can replace cheese. It is a basic recipe for vegetarians and vegans, and for children with problems like Abby (needing to avoid milk foods and cheese). It can be used to accompany potatoes, cauliflower, endives, salads, etc. Use it on open sandwiches, for picnics, with savory pancakes, and so on.

Recipe for tofu ice-cream or sherbet (four people)

Take 250 g of ripened strawberries, 250 g of apples (Golden), 125 g of tofu, a vanilla pod, a tablespoon of barley malt , a tablespoon of one of the above jams, a tablespoon of acacia honey, the juice of half a lemon, a (small) drop of essential oil of peppermint and half a cup of water.

Rinse the tofu, put it in the mixer with the lemon juice, the vanilla broken up and the half cup of water. Switch on the mixer. When it "creams" take out two tablespoons and set them aside (for decoration). Add the strawberries and apple (grated) into the mixer bowl with the "tofu cream." After mixing, place in the refrigerator and serve as an iced cream. Or place in the freezer compartment for several hours, it can be served as an ice cream. If you keep it for a few days it must be remixed to get rid of the crystallized "flakes." The small quantity of tofu cream set aside can be served as a decoration for either of these presentations.

If tofu is not used, you simply get a natural sherbet; choose fruits in season (apricots, peaches, etc.) and flavor with a drop of "organic" lemon or orange essence.

Scented summer cooler

Finally, a small recipe for summer days, highly appreciated by children: Put two tablespoons of honey into a mixer, add two drops of citrus essence (orange, lemon, tangerine, grapefruit) or of your preferred essential oil (peppermint, corn mint, bitter orange, or even rose–why not?); mix well with the honey, add half a liter of water, mix and chill. This scented water, poured into ice cube containers, can be prepared the day before and will alleviate the thirst of your children both aromatically and healthily.

Note on soy products

If I recommend tofu, this is because it is the result of a transformation process that renders the soya proteins highly digestible and easily assimilable. On the other hand, I advise the greatest caution in using soya milk. We shall revert to this at a future date, when I shall deal in greater depth with natural nutrition and give a good many other healthy and savory recipes.

SIMPLE FOOT REFLEXOLOGY AS PART OF R.A.C.
FIRST PRESENTATION OF THE Q (PSY) POINT

I understand that some readers feel skepticism, doubt or refusal reactions in response to some of our proposals. It is their right and I recognize it. This is the place where they are now and probably need to be for their internal safety. But life is a film, not a photo taken once for all. Things change and people change. When you have lived through as many coincidences or rather, as you say in English, synchronicity events, as we have in this unbelievable life, you will perhaps begin to ask yourself some questions about the existence of another reality, an upper Reality, which eventually turns out to be the Ultimate Reality, beyond the plane of physical manifestations.

If all of this were just fairy tales, New Age ideas, drug-induced hallucinations, etc., believe me, all the intelligence service institutions of the world, including the CIA and the former KGB, would not have invested so much time, money and effort in the exciting research on the power of the human spirit.

But our aim here is not in spying and ripping off secrets. It is on sharing what we have discovered and offering it to those who want to expand their natural healing capacities in a simple and efficacious way.

Foot reflexology is very well known and well-accepted in English speaking countries. France is quite delayed in this regard, but things are beginning to move forward a bit more nowadays. Reflex points exist in many parts of the body besides the feet: ears, nose (outside and inside), eyes, tongue, hands, the skull, all the joints (ankles, knees, hips, wrists, elbows, shoulders), etc. However, which of these areas is the most neglected and kept "imprisoned" almost all day long in our modern world? Yes, the feet!

In order for my patients to better understand the importance of massaging and setting free the reflex points of the feet, I use this comparison: Imagine you want to drive your car. You know that there is enough fuel in the tank, enough lubricating oil, enough cooling fluid, etc. You start the motor and you begin to move. However, you find that your car does not move at its normal speed, something is hindering it. Guess what happened? You forgot to do a simple task: release the handbrake! It has happened to me and it surely has occurred to you. Well, in the case of your body, the handbrake is in your feet. Just using essential oils on the body and forgetting to set free the points of the feet means that you will not get the full life-enhancing power of the aromatic substance! The energy is not circulating properly in the body and it is important to begin with the feet

As a matter of fact, in most cases, any practical session with us starts with releasing the reflex points of the feet. I am sure most English-speaking readers have seen the charts illustrating the reflex points of the feet. The one which is proposed here (See Photo No. 35), was not intended to show all the details, but rather to simplify the concept in order to enable you to practice this important form of foot massage in your home, with your family. As a standard practice in our clinic, we begin by warming the feet (we use a "Spectron generator," a Chinese system that rebalances the energy flow of the body).

In your home, you should have the person receiving the massage lie comfortably and you should begin the massage in a position in which you also feel comfortable. You can use an EO adapted to the treatment you wish to provide; it should be diluted in a base vegetable oil. I recommend including some oil of *Calophylium inophyllum* which also works thera-peutically (and not just as a carrier for the essential oil).

For an evening massage, some lavandin or true lavender EO is suit-able; for a day massage, Rosemary EO (camphor-cineole) is a good basic choice. Here are the steps to follow:

1. First, make "contact" and massage the whole foot with some aro-matic massage oil. Begin with the right foot and follow with the left foot.

2. Then, massage the solar plexus area on the foot, turning clockwise (See Photo No. 37).

3. Progressively increase the size of the circle until you follow the pathway of the large intestine, always clockwise. For the right foot, you go up and then horizontally from left to right; for the left foot, you continue the movement horizontally and then you go downward and you finish inward. Normally, you massage for two minutes on the right half of the bowel (on the right foot) and then you continue with a two minute mas-sage on the left half of the large intestine (on the left foot).

4. Work on the liver area, the spleen area, the stomach and pancreas areas, and on the kidney/adrenal gland area (See Photo Nos. 38, 40 and 41).

5. Proceed to the lung areas of both feet (See Photo No. 39).

6. For the genital organs, work on the point shown on the map under the heel and also on each side of the heel (See Photo No. 42).

7. The pituitary point requires a pressure with the knuckle of the index or of the thumb (See Photo No. 36).

8. For the sinuses, press on and massage the top of each of the toes. If you have acquired a glass rod (or any equivalent suitable object), it can be useful for massaging those small areas (See Photo No. 43).

It should take about 20 minutes for you to complete this full cycle for both feet.

The "Ψ" (Psy) Point

With this quick background on reflexology areas, I now want to present the discovery of an important new reflex point we call the "Q" (Psy) point. In 1988, Rose-Marie and I were doing some careful research on the reflex point of the foot. As usual, and this is a radical departure from conventional medical research, we like to experiment with new techniques on ourselves first. One day, as Rose-Marie was working on my feet, she was "attracted" to an area which, to our knowledge, had not been described as having a specific connection to, or relation to, the patient's psychological well-being.

You can see this area on the photo foot map (See Photo No. 35). It is located at the base of the big toe, on its external side, or the side facing the second toe (See Photo No. 44). Rose-Marie began to massage this point that she found was very tender and blocked (which is normal for a point which had never been treated before). She massaged these points on both feet and I remember, since the massage was performed in the evening, that it triggered a profound state a relaxation, a deep impression of "letting go" and "liberation of tensions." I fell asleep immediately afterward and during the night following this special massage, a sort of complete spiritual cleansing took place. When this area is unblocked, it is as if a hand was penetrating into the skull and was massaging the whole mass of the brain to purify it and accomplish a kind of natural and accelerated analysis or "footreflex psychotherapy."[1]

This is how the "Psy Point," as we call it now, was discovered. As often happens in our life, very soon after this discovery we had the occasion to prove its high value in an extreme case (this is what we call synchronicity):

I remember the day when Mrs L. rang me for an appointment Already on the phone, I had the feeling I was talking with someone who was among the "walking dead." There was no life left in her voice and I knew it was going to be a very special experience to meet this person. My first phone impression was totally confirmed when I saw her entering the clinic (at the time we were working 40 km south of Paris, where we spent five years before moving to the south of France in the Drôme valley).

She was a tall lady in her mid forties but what was most striking was the fact she appeared as though all that makes a human being alive had left her. There was a thin body sitting in front of me from which the part that gives real life to a human being had almost completely disappeared. Often in my teaching as well as with my patients, I like to take concrete examples, simple and understandable analogies, to make things clear. Concerning the relationship between body and soul, to keep to common terms, I put on a glove on my right hand; but, instead of fitting the glove tightly, I leave it half way off. In that case, it is obvious that even though you move your fingers, the result in terms of moving or seizing objects or doing anything creative with your fingers, will be rather poor or even impossible.

In this analogy, the glove represents the body and the hand represents the soul. The equivalent in French for the English word "soul" is "l' âme." Whereas the etymology of the word "soul," according to the English Oxford Dictionary, is a bit confusing, for Latin languages, it is quite clear. It comes from the root "Anima." In Jungian psychology, "anima" refers also to the feminine principle as present in the male subconscious and "animus" as the masculine principle present in the female subconscious; but we'll stick with the basic Latin root. The Romans created their word "anima" from the Greek language. Now what meanings were attached to this root word? Perhaps you have heard of the word "anemometer?" Some of you weather buffs certainly know the answer. For the rest, I will mention the Greek root "ανεγο" (read it "anemo") which means "wind." So, an anemometer is a measuring device for wind, specifically wind speed. Does this ring a bell? In Chapter 4, we mentioned the "wind of life" or rather the "breath of life" being breathed through the nostrils.

In the case of Mrs. L., it was as if the hand had almost left the glove. Her breathing was reduced to minimal survival level. My first appointment with her took an hour and a half, and it consisted simply in listening to her personal horror story. I will summarize it for you to help you understand how a human being can be destroyed by traumatic experiences and modern medicine's utter inability to deal with trauma from a psychological and energetic point of view. (I admire the technical work performed, but that alone is not sufficient to cure the problem. Hence the need for complementary approaches.)

Four years earlier, Mrs. L. was hosting a summer party in the garden of their home. Her fifteen-year old son was in charge of the BBQ. He felt the charcoal was not burning fast enough, so he decided to pour alcohol on it. Well, you can imagine the result of such foolishness: he was transformed into a human torch in front of his mother's eyes! He was rushed to the hospital in a desperate state of deep and extensive burning. For a whole month, his mother could only look at him behind the glass of the intensive care unit. She saw him day and night in intense pain and she prayed intensely so that his life would be spared. She said she would give her own life to see her son healed. The medical and surgical treatments managed to save him, but Mrs. L., a few months later, was diagnosed with cancer of the uterus. In a way, she was accomplishing the self fulfilling prophecy of giving her own life, and the uterus is very symbolic in this context.

Again, modern medicine and surgery did what they had to do and she was "physically cured." But what about her psychological state? She was simply left destroyed, annihilated, mentally and humanly lifeless after these two successive ordeals.

The different psychoactive drugs that she had been given, were totally incapable of working in a way that would cicatrize her deep "soul" wounds. The living proof of this inability was her present condition of bare survival. After having heard her horror story in minute detail, I was myself almost overcome. I know they teach in theoretical psychotherapy you should not get involved in the patient's situation, but this time, it had gone too far!

So, we talked with Rose-Marie and we decided to begin to treat her two days later. This was a unique opportunity for Rose-Marie to confirm her serendipitous inspiration concerning the "Psy" point. Mrs L. agreed to undertake this exclusive treatment, and two days later, she was lying on the couch, waiting for her revival experience.

So, what I will tell you now will sound incredible. I can't force you to believe it, but I assure you it is the plain truth, no more, no less. Rose-Marie performed the Reflexology treatment on the feet. She was eager to discover what massage of this Psy point would trigger in the case of such a deeply shocked person. As a matter of fact, the Psy points on her feet proved to be sensitive to such an extreme degree, that it was simply impossible even to touch them, let alone to exert slight pressure! In fact, a kind of roll of flesh had been formed over those past four years and the day to dissolve it had now arrived. The only way to tackle the treatment was to work with a subtle and most gentle "effleurage," i.e. a way of touching that is so light that you normally feel almost nothing. In Mrs L.'s case, even this "angel's touch" created pain!

Rose-Marie spent 20 minutes doing this "effleurage" procedure on the right Psy point and 10 minutes for all the other toes. The same treatment was done on the left foot: 20 minutes of effleurage on the Psy point and 10 minutes for the other toes. This represented one hour spent only on the toes. The 20 minutes spent on each big toe were not consecutive; Rose-Marie worked on the other toes in between. If not it would have been too painful. The total time spent on the feet amounted to one hour and a half.

This first session triggered immediately an immense change from a psychological point of view. The week after, we saw a lady returning to a normal state of life. A second session was performed, and this time it was possible to exert a stronger pressure on the Psy points of the big toes.

After the second session, the transformation was impressive, morally as well as physically. A month later, Mrs L. was the person she used to be before the first accident. Even though her daughter had a serious car accident, she told us that she had been in a completely different state of mind that enabled her to react positively and efficaciously. The allopathic psycho-active drugs were progressively decreased until they were no longer needed. Two months later, she decided to open a business and to return to a fully normal and successful life!

We have had since that time many experiences with the inside of the big toe! It has become for us a staple reflex point whenever deep psychological trauma has left its mark both mentally and physically.

We remember quite well another case that occurred around the same time. A lady in her forties had consulted us for a skin problem on her face (redness and pimples that made her face quite inelegant). The problem had begun one month ago at the occasion of a serious conflict with her sixteen year old son. Knowing that, she received the 'unblocking massage' on the Psy point of the big toe as the main treatment. Two days later, almost all the pimples and the redness had vanished away!

We have had a large number of real and surprising experiences with the Psy point. When we give training seminars, we show in a practical way how to proceed. However, each therapist can locate this sore area and begin to treat it with the basic knowledge given in this book. Foot reflexology is so important in natural medicine and in natural holistic health care that we had to introduce it from this first book, with our specific contribution.[27]

The reason we schedule couple or family appointments, instead of just a single member of the family is to show them how they can continue their treatments at home. This is the way to obtain the best results: one session a week with the therapist and in between, daily sessions to be practiced at home.

GUIDELINES FOR HEALTHY BREATHING

Life begins with our first cry and ends with our last breath, A characteristic feature of human beings is their capacity to control their breath, its rhythm and its amplitude.

Many books have been written about the importance of breathing and its influence from a physical and psychological approach. Unfortunately, there is a long distance between theory and practice. When Yoga teachers consult us, I check their breathing expertise and I often find that even they have difficulties in breathing with their tummy, i.e. with a full movement of their diaphragm.

As a professional singer, I was trained by Madame Walter who was at a time Line Renaud's tutor (Line Renaud is well known in Las Vegas). I have used breathing techniques for more than 20 years. I was put directly on the right track, educated first and foremost in abdominal breathing. With the practice of Yoga, Tai Chi, Qui Kong, moving meditation, Biosynergy, I met many teachers and I experimented a lot on myself and then on patients.

When a baby breathes, it is always through the abdomen. If we want to reconnect with our roots, we need to relearn this abdominal way of breathing.

I have learned many breathing techniques, but I found that abdominal breathing is the best way to work from a therapeutic point of view in order to get rid of stress, to eliminate mental parasites, to get well-rooted with our feet on the earth and at the same time mentally open to the Universe, like a wire that connects both poles. I have stated that people know complex things, they forget simple things. Therefore, I ask them to forget a little bit about the difficult things that they seem to master and to go back to basics, to the primordial simplicity, to the essential.

I have found the same pattern with breathing as with nutrition. The mind regulates breathing and breathing in its turn controls body movement. In practice, here is what I advise you to do:

Begin by standing up, bare foot, well rooted on the ground, letting go of all tensions.

This is a prelude to the breathing exercise itself. Both fists are applied on the solar plexus area: you open your arms and extend them wide apart while exhaling used air and used thoughts. This procedure is done three times, breathing as usual. You end up with crossed arms in front of the body.

In this first book, I prefer to teach one main exercise, rather than to ask too much and get no practical results.

It can be practiced while standing up, or sitting or lying. First, put both hands on the lower abdomen and begin by breathing out through your mouth. The tummy becomes hollow (at least in thought) until it touches the spine. Mentally picture the bad things being expelled and neutralized in a river, in a lake, in the sea, in the mountain atmosphere, whatever you choose as a mental picture.

1. Keep the fingers on the lower abdomen and breathe in while visualizing the blue or the orange color. This breathing in lasts two counts (you count one, two) and be careful to keep the breath in the tummy, do not expand the thoracic area.

2. Hold the color in your mind and the air in the tummy for four counts (you count one, two, three, four).

3. Then you exhale for four counts, and

4. Then you remain with empty lungs for four counts.

Even if you cannot practice the prelude, this simple breathing exercise will be whole by itself. This breathing exercise can be done before each meal (one minute is enough, and it makes a big difference), when coming back from work (and in that case, it is better to do it lying down) or when you feel tired or stressed. In the work place, you may perform it with discretion whenever you need to recover strength and calmness.

When you work hard studying for an exam or any intellectual task, it is good to practice it every hour.

My conclusion: now with natural nutrition, foot reflex massage and good breathing, you have a powerful triad upon which you can build your own health.

The next step will be…to sing
With all wishes of full blossoming

Rose-Marie PÉNOËL

Footnotes:

27. It might be that other therapists have discovered the same area and have riot published their result or perhaps have published it in articles or books which we have not yet seen: in that case. they can get in touch with our distributor and we are more than happy to exchange information and experiences and mention them in future writings.

CHAPTER 6

QUESTIONS FOR
DR. PÉNOËL

I want the last chapter of Part II to be similar to an open Q & A session as it often takes place during or near the end of my seminars. Remember that this book is a basic introduction to a whole concept and method. Clearly in this book we have focused heavily on respiratory and ENT problems. One reason for this is because of the introductory, prototype case of little Abby, but it is also because EOs are particularly effective in this arena and because conventional medicine truly needs better solutions than it now has to achieve real healing efficiency in this area.

EOs can be implemented, with similar success in practically every other field of medicine. But this introductory book is already very rich in new information and applications for a good start with your family. If I had to put everything in a single book, it would be impossible to produce it and to sell it.

Now let's start our Q & A session and I will list the most common questions I am asked at my seminars. For consistency and in the context of my July, 1998, seminar in Salt Lake City I will answer these questions as if I were in front of an American audience. But you may transpose it to whatever location you wish. These questions tend to be the same no matter where I go.

The text has only received minimal correction, since you have me facing you talking directly to you in my own English. So, forgive the imperfections, but the heart is there and it gives a touch of greater reality to the book.

Question No. 1: Dr Pénoël, can you tell us how you perceive the role of EOs and aromatherapy in the management of cancerous diseases?

DP: Well, you begin with a tough question! First of all, I want you to understand that this is a highly complex subject which obviously cannot be properly covered in a simple and short answer. When you think of the treatment of any disease, what you have in your mind is a curative treatment. Then, you should remember the English saying that states: "An ounce of prevention is worth a pound of cure." As a matter of fact, the modern civilized world that we have created is, by itself, the perfect example, on a planetary scale, of a monstrous cancer.

From a global and systemic approach, you can look at a cancerous cell as a cell that has lost all sense of respect for the other cells around it, and for the whole organism, You could describe its attitude as:

"Me, only me, and to hell with everyone else!"

Well, such gross selfishness will end up over time destroying the host organism and therefore the tumor itself. But in between, what intense ordeals and sufferings will have been produced! From a single cell that becomes so crazy that it no longer respects its host and its companions, a tumor is formed, which continually grows larger, and the whole organism can be invaded through metastasis sent from the tumor to other parts of the body.

If you take this picture of an individual cancer and enlarge this perception to the whole planet, you will clearly perceive that, from an ecological point of view, mankind, with its chemical craziness and its overall destruction of the ecosystem, represents the cancer of planet earth. With our collective behavior we are literally sawing the branch on which we are sitting.

If you remember in the Bible, it is written: "He who lives by the sword will perish by the sword" (Matthew 26:52). This can be transposed for our time: "He who lives by chemical products will perish because of chemical products." Nowadays, if you happen to visit a typical farm (and generally the farmer is not willing to let you easily discover the hidden side of his farm), you would be appalled and disgusted to see first hand the amazing amount of deadly chemical "stuff" that is stored in his barn, waiting to be poured on the fields, and to be sprayed on the plants and on the trees. It is all labeled with poison signs. In this case, it is painfully true! If a farmer has not made a deliberate choice to practice organic farming, you can be sure that he is highly involved in chemical agro-business. The same applies with the breeding of farm animals, be it for milk, eggs or meat.

In the same way, any conventional MD, who has not made a personal choice to study natural medicine in addition to his standard training, can only give you a chemically-oriented therapeutic answer.

So the chemical industry has two huge, almost fathomless, pockets. In the first pocket, it accumulates the benefits from planetary agro-business; and because we become sick with the chemical products we breathe, drink and eat, we seek advice from the medical system. And what do we get? More chemical drugs to pour into our bodies. And where do the benefits go? Well, they rush into a huge, fathomless second pocket, the one linked to the highly refined petrochemistry industry called the pharmaceutical business. (I have many pharmacist friends in France who agree with me on this; hence, the alternative choices that have become available.)

This is just to mention the chemical side. But radiations, infections and in particular viral aggressions, psychological traumas and many other contributing factors work in synergy or with a cumulative and multiplicative effect, so that what astonishes me is not the large number of cancers, but rather the fact that some of us still manage to escape cancer! Mind you, if all those who have died from car accidents, heart attacks and many other diseases had lived longer, they would probably have enriched the statistics of deaths by cancer.

What I wish you to understand is that everyday, I, you, your friends, all of us–we create a certain number of cancerous cells. It is part of the game of life, that's all. Thank God, our immune system is alert and awake all the time and cancerous cells are arrested like policemen or soldiers would do with any enemy or crazy person and they are destroyed. (But of course I am not suggesting here to "destroy" the human persons, rather to make them change their behavior.)

At the end of this day for instance, 100 cells have turned crazy in my body; those 100 potential or already cancerous cells will have been recognized and eliminated. Final result = 0 cancerous cells left. If only one cell manages to escape the persistence and perspicacity of our immune system, that single cell will multiply rapidly until it can make a tumor comprised of billions of cancerous cells. If you begin to change your life for the better, you will definitely decrease the risks of developing a cancer.

I do not say that those who live a healthy life will never have cancer. I simply state, from a probability and statistical point of view, that cancers are less frequent when we follow the laws of natural health. And this is not just one view of the mind, since it has been proven, in the U.S., when checking the percentage of colon cancer in large groups like the Mormons and the Seventh Day Adventists, whose habits (in particular eating habits) are quite different from the typical American way of Life. From a practical point of view, my advice is simple and clear:

First of all, understand that you are the one most responsible for having or not having cancer. On the prevention side of the treatment, you must take charge of your own lifestyle. In particular, if you still smoke, quitting smoking is the first step to undertake! Aromatherapy can help you with calming essential oils and respiratory purifying oils. But the most important part begins in your mind. Let me tell you a story, a true one.

During my medical studies, I happened to work in the hospital of Montreuil (in the close vicinity of Paris), which was considered at the time as a rather poor area, mainly populated, as you say in English, with "blue collars." Well, may be you won't believe me, but here is what I saw in the ENT surgical ward off the hospital. A guy, in his fifties, who had smoked since he was a teenager, had had his larynx removed for cancer. He had a hole in the front of his neck with a tube inserted in it. So, he was not breathing through his mouth or his nostrils, but directly through his trachea. For obvious physical reasons, it was impossible for this person to smoke. You really think so? Well, remain well seated, because what I saw might disturb you. It let me in a state of dismay! You guess what I am going to tell you? Yes, you're perfectly right: I saw the poor tobacco-addicted guy inserting the end of the cigarette at the entrance of the tube, blocking around the void space and aspiring with delight the deadly gaseous substance!! Mind you, having reached this stage, he might not have a lot to lose. Why not insert the cigarette directly into the bronchial system? Apart from the burning risk, it would prove even more convenient!

Can you visualize yourself, if you're a smoker, reaching such an extreme and desperate degree of addiction? You might think that you are not so much addicted? Well, just prove it! You know what? The very next time you think of lighting up a cigarette, simply decide to leave it in its packet. If you do that, believe me, you can already be and feel very proud of this first little step. And each little step following that one will bring you a sincere joy to regain control that will far outweigh the little destructive pleasures that come from not smoking.

One thing is sure: you cannot, at the same time, play host to God and the devil. When Dr. Jekyll was Dr. Jekyll, he was not Mr. Hyde, and vice versa. If essential oils, which represent life, become really integrated into your life, it will become more and more difficult for tobacco to remain your worst "friend."

I know that most smokers do not like to smell Eucalyptus oil. Well, Eucalyptus is precisely what will help to purify the respiratory system from decades of pulmonary poisoning! So, when some teachers insist that you should only use the EOs that seem olfactively pleasant, I think this is too narrow a view.

Maybe if we were 100% healthy and "saints," such an approach would apply more logically. But in our internally and externally polluted reality, things are not that simple! Sometimes, it is the very EO that is disliked that represents a corrective factor for the patient. Then, the art of the therapist is to learn how to apply it in an acceptable way. The penetration through the sole of the feet is generally the easiest and least aggressive way to do it. If both partners in a couple smoke, it is advisable to undertake quitting together. A consultation with an aromatherapist (or other natural health professional) might be of a great help. And remember to drink a lot and to take some supplements (natural vitamins B and C, in particular) in order to help the detoxification process. I prefer in any case the implementation of a holistic approach in a natural health program, including intensive and regular aromatherapy, don't just focus on quitting smoking. The quitting smoking will be included as a key element in a broad program and with a much less intense effort than in the restricted approach. And do not forget that coffee, tea, chocolate, cola and foods rich in refined sugar are also, in this overall context, considered potentially addictive substances.

I have seen patients who quit smoking tell me the following apparently paradoxical adventure: "You know Dr Pénoël, when I was a smoker, I had from time to time some coughing. Now that I have quit smoking, it seems to me that I cough and reject more mucus than before!" Well, in fact, this is understandable and logical. Now that the body has a real chance to purify itself, particularly the mucus membranes of the bronchial tree, it takes advantage of the opportunity in an accelerated way. The application of the basic respiratory blends that I described before is quite useful for helping this necessary "atonement phase." Do not think that I am an extreme "puritan." If smoking two or three cigarettes a day is simply for you a way to relax, and if you do not feel addicted to tobacco, the risk is low. But you could invent a different way to get rid of your tensions, couldn't you!

From the vast and intense foot reflexology experience acquired through practice by Rose-Marie and I, I can tell you that setting free the Psy Point of your big toes (I can almost feel it from here!) can prove very helpful in strengthening the nervous system and in helping your psychological resolve to eliminate your addictive habit. In any case, one day or another you will become an ex-smoker. Therefore, why not decide to begin today, instead of procrastinating all the time? Millions have done it and are so happy and proud of their newly acquired freedom, I bet you can do it too. When? Well, the sooner the better... And why not here and now? Remember that "to decide" comes from the Latin and means "to cut" (like with a scissors). Seize that packet of poison in your pocket and take each cigarette in its turn and cut it twice in two, with a scissors, in the length and in the middle. With this symbolic gesture of liberation you will have begun recovering your will power over what was your former deadly habit.

You see, it is not as impossible as you imagined it would be!

Concerning the nutritional aspect you will find hundreds of books about natural nutrition. The most important is to work from a long term perspective. You are not following a quick fix program as the ones described in magazines for losing weight before summer comes. You are reforming your lifestyle, including what you eat and how you eat! This can only be done in the context of a family-accepted reform. Health food shops, be it in the U.S., in Canada, in Great Britain, in Australia or in New-Zealand provide a large range of nice, natural, tasty foods and trained staff who will be happy to guide you in the first steps. If you buy from the market or local growers, you can still find some sensible small farmers who respect the earth and themselves (many cases of professional cancer are known among farmers who use chemical pesticides).

Regular exercise, bringing oxygen into your body and helping to relax the mind, should be part of your program. The most important objective, in a long-term perspective, is to obtain physical pleasure and mental joy from the sports in which you engage.

Including essential oils in a regular way in your life and learning not to jump straight into antibiotics for every kind of infection, will keep your immune system in a state of alertness and vigilance that represents the best guarantee for eliminating "crazy selfish cells."

In a more subtle vein, using EO for relaxation and the release of nervous and psychological tensions can contribute significantly to your overall state of balance. People addicted to Prozac® and similar kinds of drugs are not helping their immune systems, exactly like those who are taking antibiotics all the time (often these are the same people!). French patients and their doctors sadly hold the world's absolute record for the highest use of psychoactive pharmaceutical drugs, and from our perspective in natural medicine and aromatherapy, we know that there are so many natural ways to help them, if only they would accept it. Last, but not least, turning to EO and to aromatherapy from a perspective of obtaining pleasure and joy generates the secretion of "internal healing substances" (endorphins and the like) that will boost one's overall immunity. Make your immune cells "sing and dance" everyday that God gives you to live. This is certainly the secret of long-lasting health.

Creating psychological and spiritual harmony in your life is definitely a most important task. Without it, all the efforts made to improve your physical health might be in vain. In this respect, you can think of Saint Augustin's words: "Love, and do what you like." Of course, this has to be understood in the deepest meaning of the verb "love."

When cancer is already present, can aromatherapy help and how? Well, there are hundreds of kinds of cancers with different stages of growth and invasion. Patients with cancer are treated in hospitals with modem means of action: In general chemotherapy, surgery, radiotherapy, etc, The role of aromatherapy and other natural therapies can be a determining factor in helping the conventional treatments. So, normally, we have here a perfect example of complementarity.

In most cases, aromatic molecules have not been created to kill cells! On the contrary, they are helping life and regeneration. So, it is important

to have the patient understand that he will increase his survival and strug-
gling capacity with alternative medicine, including aromatherapy. This
being clearly stated, it is true that almost all therapists have had extreme
cases where the patient had been abandoned by modern medicine as
being "beyond all hope" and essential oils (included in a holistic program)
have shown incredible results. This is not a reason to embark into foolish
actions. Those cases help us perceive that we have a lot to discover in this
fantastic world of aromatic plants, but it will have to be done in conjunction with modern research and not in opposition to it.

At this stage, you will have to seek advice from natural therapists, if
possible also trained in aromatherapy, and/or with trained aromatherapists,
who will work in parallel with your surgeon and the medical specialists
who provide you with the best of their knowledge and know-how.

Remember that prevention remains our first priority. Be aware that the
kind of natural lifestyle that you read about in all the books can also help
you in avoiding most of the other degenerative diseases of modern society,
the kind that you are heading to if you spend your daily eating time in
those American-originated and now world-invading, health-robbing, fast
food restaurants.

**Question No. 2: Dr Pénoël, how do you approach allergic diseases
with aromatherapy?**

DP: Here again, the subject is highly complex and I cannot give you a
magical quick fix for any kind of allergy. First, you should know that
allergies are classified into specific categories and it is worthwhile to obtain,
at the very least, a clear conventional diagnosis of your own case. This
does not mean that in natural medicine we share the same view as conventional doctors, but we always appreciate having access to as much
scientific data as possible.

From my natural medical approach, I can already tell you that we usually tackle the allergic problems with an in-depth nutritional audit. Whether
expressed on the skin or in the respiratory system, allergies are seen from
the naturopathic viewpoint as efforts by the body to expel toxic elements
which basically come from what is absorbed in the digestive system.

The classic examples we have of this reality come from children who
have eczema and are taken by their mothers to the GP or to the derma-

tologist. Generally, the child will end up with a sort of cortisone ointment to be applied, and of course, no serious nutritional advice (at least with French dermatologists or allopathic GPs). The quick fix solution might seem miraculous in the beginning. But how many children have later become asthmatic, which is worse than having eczema. In reality, asthma is like the internalization of eczema, as if it had been simply masked, hidden on the external part of the body and re-channeled inside.

Generally, dairy products and wheat will have to be monitored and probably totally suppressed for a while, while providing healthy nutritional advice and giving natural treatments. You already know that essential oils have to be used with great caution with allergic patients and those cases should be treated by natural therapists also trained in aromatherapy. If essential oils are to be applied for soothing the itching and the skin irritation, they should be of the highest possible quality, organically certified or wild, and used in very low concentration.

Because I know you like concrete advice, I will give you a possible oil blend to try along with a change in eating habits. There is a wonderful essential oil that is produced in the Drôme valley (they are distilling it now, in June-July), and it is extremely expensive (more than Rose). It is the genuine EO extracted from *Melissa officinalis* (Lemon balm in English). The yield is one of the lowest you can imagine. However, if you can obtain the organically certified EO of lemon balm, you will only use a minute amount of it. To reinforce its action I combine it with EO of German chamomile *(Maricaria recutita)* and EO of wild true (high mountain) lavender.

The carrier oil should be a top quality one, like borage or evening primrose oil (rich in GLA). For 20 ml to 30 ml of carrier oil, you can count half a drop (a "French drop" from a pipette) to one drop of lemon balm EO, two drops of German chamomile and three drops of the best lavender EO you can find. So even if these EOs have a high price, the total amount that is used is quite small.

For small children, I advise parents to apply this blend very gently with a thin silk painting brush on the irritated and itchy areas. This has given me good results, again included in the context of a holistic and nutritional approach.

Asthma is an even more complex problem and normally we spend a lot of time during a first appointment with this one. Therefore I have to say again, that none of these situations has a quick fix solution. Still, I know that sometimes very simple measures can prove quite helpful, at least in a first stage, like the care that would be provided by emergency help on the road by an emergency mechanic before being taken into the garage for complete diagnosis and repair.

With asthmatic children, the basic EO that I use is Niaouli (generally from Madagascar). In laboratory conditions, we have access to a very large number of EOs and the formulations are created according to three complementary levels of action, namely matter, energy and information. Here, the aim is to remain simple and practical in a natural self-help context. Here is one such basic formulation for use with asthma. It is only one of many. There is nothing magic about it.

EO of Niaouli	15 ml
EO of Canadian Balsam Fir	2 ml
EO of Carraway	1 ml
EO of Eucalyptus dives	1 ml
EO of Tarragon	0.5 ml
EO of Lemon scented gum (Eucalyptus citriodora)	0.5 ml
EO of Lemongrass (Cymbopogon flexuosus)	0.5 ml
EO of Peppermint	0.5 ml

If infections usually accompany the allergy/asthma as a complication, some EO of Tea Tree Oil (2 ml) should be added to this formula.

In the case of a five-year old child, I would recommend applying three drops of the blend on the lung area of each foot, once or twice a day. Quantities can be increased for larger patients. Tarragon EO is known to be endowed with anti-allergic properties. In France, it is very difficult to use EOs rich in anethole: fennel, anis and Chinese star anise. In other countries, this is not the case. You could add 1 ml of one of these EOs to the blend to increase the antispasmodic action. Here we want a quick penetration and the blend is applied neat. Also, if some foot massage is possible, the blend can be added to a carrier oil, at the usual concentration of English Style Aromatherapy.

A complex formulation can entail other EOs chosen according to deep biochemical understanding of their components. Last but not least a very common problem, not so serious but quite irritating if you have it, is hay-fever. Just three days ago, a patient phoned me and told me that from the first day she tried the following blend, she had stopped sneezing and weeping and being irritated. So, I want you to benefit from this potential help. I do not say it is a cure-all for any hay fever, but it deserves to be tried honestly, if not for a complete cure, at least for a certain degree of relief.

Tarragon EO	5 ml
Scotch Pine EO	1.5 ml
Peppermint EO	0.5 ml
Roman Chamomile EO	two (English) drops

Now, I want to give some recommendations about the quality of EOs in this case.

Organic EO of tarragon exists (it is grown in Spain and organically certified according to the European control system). But I must recognize that it is not easily available. If you can get it organic, it is the best; if not, you will have to make do with what is available to you. If you cannot get Tarragon EO, you can try Tropical Basil (methyl chavicol type). But tarragon would be the first choice. Now, Tropical Basil is more easily available as organically grown (it is produced in Vietnam but other countries have begun to produce it organically). Peppermint and Roman Chamomile are normally available as organically certified. With Scotch pine (Pinus sylvestris). the situation needs to be clarified. Most "recreational fragrancing," types of companies would simply sell "pine oil," which could be almost anything produced as a byproduct of the conifer timber industry! So, be very careful! Once you have smelled the highly subtle scent of genuine EO of Scotch Pine, you will forever remember it and no longer confuse it with any other.

You should know that, at the production level, a conifer EO produced for therapeutic aromatherapy costs up to ten times more (and sometimes twenty times more) than the timber industry's "aromatic byproducts." If you cannot be sure of the quality of the EO you get, leave it out of the formula.

The way to use this blend is similar to what we do with tea tree oil in a case of sore throat: a trace of it is applied on the tongue, several times per day, according to the symptoms. A trace can also be inhaled using a drop or two on a tissue, always beginning with caution in case of nasal allergies.

So, you now have something to begin with, but remember that the problem will probably require more in-depth management and you should certainly make some changes in your eating habits, beginning with decreasing (or stopping for a while) all that comes from cow's (milk, cream, butter, cheese). Just taking this basic step, in and of itself, will make a significant difference.

My last piece of advice is that in most cases of allergies, there is deep inside a pathological flora that needs to be corrected. If at this point you have learned how to avoid "the antibiotics response" and consider treating your family and yourself with integral aromatherapy, it will be a great achievement for building your future health assets!

Question No. 3: Dr Pénoël, can you give us some advice about autoimmune diseases?

DP: Again, a tough question to answer briefly, but I can give you here also some basic facts. First, I want to tell you something important. It concerns Abby. Well, imagine we had not been granted our Australian visas, we would never have met Abby. She would have stayed imprisoned in the conventional medical system. Maybe the surgery and the antibiotic bombarding would have seemed, after more years, to "solve" the problem.... (I believe such a notion is a total illusion.)

In reality, there was simply no way apart from natural and aromatic medicine to help Abby. What I know through clinical experience is that after many years, patients who have had a history of ENT infections treated by antibiotics, often–at the occasion of a psychological trauma (bereavement after a death, divorce, emotional shock, etc)–manifest an autoimmune disease known as rheumatoid arthritis. Of course, a joint specialist consulting with a patient aged 40 never makes the connection between that disease and something that happened during her childhood, but the real and deep causes lie there.

The process develops like this: it begins with repeated infections treated repeatedly with antibiotics. After several years of such "dysbiosis" (= bad life), allergic problems come to the forefront. Then, cortisone drugs are prescribed in the treatment. The last stage along this degenerative pathway is taken when an internal autoimmune disease appears.

As part of a modern campaign to increase "craziness" in our immune systems, we have a big problem in France with an intense program of vaccinations (immunizations) that are not always well-accepted in the bodies of some of the participants. Millions of French children have been required to be immunized against hepatitis B virus. The campaign was so intense that the laboratory who manufactures the vaccines had an ad (to recruit more financial participation) that said: "whenever a child gets immunized, our shareholders benefit!" We know many cases of children or teenagers who have had adverse reactions, sometimes quite serious ones. My dentist's daughter received these immunizations and shortly after, her kidneys began to be attacked by auto- antibodies (antibodies wrongly programmed to destroy the healthy cells in the body!). She has been told that she will have to receive cortisone treatments for the rest of her life! For the government, these incidents have no weight upon their bureaucratic decisions. But for the patient and the parents, what a tragedy...

You might have heard about the awful scandal surrounding the use of contaminated blood (by AIDS virus) used for blood transfusions in France. You can easily imagine that the main priority in this case, was a financial one, far above any alleged "health concern." Events like these almost make you think we are in a war with our the medical system that is supposed to help us!

What I want you to understand, basically, is very profound and very simple: it is that modem, scientific medicine actually creates its future patients by the inappropriate therapeutic actions it undertakes. And auto-immune diseases are yet another consequence of this destructive cycle. So, as with cancer, first we think of prevention through lifestyle, integrating essential oils in our daily health maintenance program and learning to use them intensively when required. When the auto-immune disease is already present, treatment depends of course on what stage the patient is in. To see a patient at the very onset of rheumatoid arthritis is one thing, but to see her after thirty years of cortisone treatments with joints that have been destroyed, is a completely different challenge.

It is true that we sometimes see situations where EOs have an almost miraculous effect. In his last book, Dr. Gary Young quotes a case of lupus where, after an application of a blend containing Frankincense EO, the patient was totally transformed and apparently became symptom-free. Case histories like this one do exist in aromatherapy (and in other natural therapies as well).

Mr Haim Schloss, from Tel Aviv, attended my training on "The intensive and internal use of EOs" given in England at Shirley Price Institute. When he went back to Israel, a female patient who had a severe case of Crohn's disease (an autoimmune disease against the cells of the intestine) was about to receive an operation. On the day before entering the hospital, she asked Mr Schloss if he could do something for her. He used the kind of formula that I teach as "general and overall anti-infectious" and gave it to her in an appropriate form for internal intake.

As strange as it might appear, the lady felt such an improvement that she decided to cancel the operation! I am pleased to learn about such cases but, at the same time, I do not want any suffering patient to think that instantaneous cures are obtained all the time. What we see here is related to a phenomenon known in physics as "resonance" and from the point of view of "energy medicine," we can understand better the occurrence of such healings. So, we do not like to speak of "miracles," in the supernatural meaning attached to this word (the Church itself is extremely strict about the term "miracle"). What I can tell you is that the pathological flora inside the bowels plays an important role in the continuation of autoimmune diseases. I remember a patient who came for a colonic irrigation. She had rheumatoid arthritis. After her cleansing session, she stated that over a period of three weeks her pain had almost totally disappeared. In another case, for a serious inflammatory process in the eye, for which ophthalmologists would generally prescribe cortisone drops, a colonic irrigation and some more natural techniques resulted in a major improvement in the situation. Can you imagine the reaction of the specialists stating that the eye inflammation had disappeared and learning that it happened mainly by cleansing the body!

Another example that was striking concerns a doctor's wife who had rheumatoid arthritis and who, advised to do so by her physiotherapist, took an aromatic bath with EO of tropical basil. She was an extremely sensitive and receptive person. This aromatic bath brought her a surprising relief of her joints inflammation.

I quote these examples to show that with some patients we see extraordinary reactions take place. They do exist. But it is not always so easy in every case. In cases of rheumatoid arthritis, it is important to ask the patient if she/he can remember what was the very first joint that began the destructive process. An EO that several patients have told me brought them good relief is peppermint EO. Generally, the pain being intense, they apply the EO neat on the area of the joint. It is important to apply the peppermint EO on this first joint also. In most cases, a complete natural health program has to be undertaken. Such a program should ideally be implemented in an integrated aromatic center. So, maybe you would like me to expand on this concept as part of a global vision for the future?

Question No. 4: Yes, Dr Pénoël, tell us how you foresee the evolution of aromatherapy in a worldwide perspective and what are your objectives?

DP: I think this is a good question for ending this Q & A session on an exciting note. In the Bible it is written: "Where, there is no vision, the people perish." (Proverbs 29:18) It is crucial for all of us to visualize, individually and collectively, the harmonious future we want to create. One thing is now certain and unavoidable: EO will occupy an ever-increasing role in global health maintenance programs. The medical profession, followed by the pharmaceutical profession, will be forced to pay greater attention to the world of plants and in particular to essential oils.

The importance of the French contribution in this regard is to speak in a language that conventional doctors understand, namely, the molecular approach to EOs. I am not saying, and this must be clear between us, that EOs should be reduced to nothing more than the matter-molecular aspect! But if you come to an MD or any medical specialist and talk a language which is not theirs, the "rejection reaction" will be almost instantaneous. If I send you a computer file written in a certain program and your computer can only read files in a different format, you will simply see on your screen strange signs and from time to time a few incoherent words.

If, in contrast, your approach is primarily based on the molecular nature of the properties and the actions of aromatic molecules, you can expect a better reception, provided, of course, the person you are talking to is a honest and open person. In my last book in French, I described in detail the three categories of persons with whom I would never waste my precious time. The flimsy person, the hypocritical one and the bad faith one. There is a fourth category, the worst, but at least you know clearly their position: the cynical one, who recognizes that you are right, but who does not care at all, since he/she is too absorbed in the 'grossly uncivil system' in which he/she is actively involved. That could well be the case of the president of a tobacco company who knows only too well the number of smokers he sends prematurely to the cemetery. (By the way, I heard yesterday on the news that a huge fire has been triggered in Kenya, destroying a vast area, and they said it was probably triggered by a cigarette carelessly thrown by a smoker. Tobacco is a disaster for the environment just as it is for the body.)

My most important mission now is a teaching and training one. Writing books and giving training seminars for very large groups is my priority, Training large groups of therapists is the best way for me to provide treatments, indirectly, to a vast number of patients.

It is also a mission to help people take charge of their own health, inside the home, through the proper use of EOs and other natural means. This is a major priority for the transition years we are about to experience. In this perspective, I think that different sorts of "Integrated Aromatic Centers" can be conceived and created. Ideally, the prototype of such a center would utilize the proficiencies of three professionals: an MD, a naturopath and a person trained in integral aromatherapy (this could be a nurse).

It could begin with out-patient care centers and evolve toward real clinical organizations for in-patient care. For difficult and chronic cases, such an environment represents the best choice. I think that some medical Institutions and hospitals are beginning to accept the idea that essential oils can be used in a medical setting, in particular under the direction of "enlightened nurses."

This growth process must be accompanied with extensive programs for growing aromatic plants in an organic way and distilling them for aromatherapeutic purposes instead of "recreational fragrancing."

Two weeks ago, I met a Norwegian lady involved in aromatherapy in her country. Ann Helen Lundestad had visited us two years ago and I had insisted at that time that they should begin to grow aromatic plants in her country and distill them. Besides, their huge forests of conifers, continuously harvested for lumber and paper, are ideal for producing EO of high quality. And she was proud to announce to me that the first Norwegian EO had just been produced. To me, helping the development of this agricultural side of aromatherapy is extremely rewarding.

We need to learn to make better use of the floral waters, and many techniques that I have developed (and that will be presented in further books) are well suited for high quality floral waters. The most important part of my task, and the most difficult, is to calm down the fierce competitive state of mind in the aromatherapy world, at all levels. May be you will say I am a dreamer, but, as they say in a well known English song, "I'm not the only one..."

I know that we have to learn from each other and I see myself more as a coach to help you develop the best of your capacities. And if you followed the 1998 World Cup Tournament, you saw clearly the major role played by a good coach, especially with the French team! Having reached a point of excellent physical condition and proficiency, what makes the winning difference between two opposing teams? Mainly the psychological conditioning; the willingness to win. The big difference for us on an individual level is that we have no opponents apart from the "bad side" inside ourselves.

Therefore, in every book you read that is written by me, you will always find the same structure, with theoretical reflection, practical use, technical applications and pervading all the pages, a spirit that is based on a sense of community, civil behavior and ecological awareness. I want again to express my feelings of gratitude, respect and admiration for your dedicated and untiring work. I want to share with you, since we talk of "perspective," a sentence that Dr. Wayne Dyer has repeated on many occasions in his most inspiring teachings (each word is important, you can meditate and ponder their meaning). It comes from the writings of Henry David Thoreau:

"If one advances confidently in the direction of his/her own dreams, and endeavors to live the life which he/she has imagined, he/she will meet with a success unexpected in common hours." And why not create a common dream and advance together in its direction?

A planetary dream, where "genuine civility" will be at the core of all our relationships, with ourselves, with others and with the whole

Biosphere? It is now in the heart of millions of us, and everyday we can make a little part of the dream become a reality.

This is my wish for all of us and for the future generations.

Thank you and may you receive all the blessings you deserve from the "Higher Power."

Dr. Daniel Pénoël
July 6, 1998

CONCLUSION

*D*ear reader, with this first publication in English we have started on our journey together together. We have been introduced to Abby, we have discovered fundamental principles, we have become fascinated by aromatic plants and their high quality extracts, we have learned simple and effective ways to care for ourselves and have noted a number of techniques rich in promise and fertile in "treasures of health." We've also received a brief apprenticeship in healthy and flavorsome recipes from Rose-Marie. I feel sure you are looking forward to the next installment of these adventures and discoveries.

The future of this collection is in your hands. If you want to further this Aromatic Revolution, make those around you aware of their responsibility and the need for them to take their into their own hands, the responsibility for their own health and that of their family members. The complete rewriting of this book's second section in two weeks has brought me new insights and helped to clarify my research teaching mission. It has also made me acutely aware of the direction my activity should take over the decisive years we are all going to live through in this transition to the 21st century.

In conclusion I should like to give some advice from long experience with my patients and share with you a few thoughts that are dear to me.

The most valuable advice I have to give is this: be confident, and above all, persevere! Years or even decades of "life out of sync with the Principles of Life" cause damage which cannot be erased overnight as if by magic.[28] If essential oils and natural medicine methods often achieve remarkable and impressive results, it must be understood that work over a long period is needed to fully transform a chronic health problem. Twenty-five years of cigarette smoking, leading a sedentary life, swallowing industrial food and treating oneself with synthetic medicines to camouflage the real causes of this "bad life" need at least a year's clean-up to give the body a real chance for regeneration. In any natural care program, therapeutic-grade essential oils greatly accelerate this total purification and energizing phase of a devitalized body. But treatment must proceed all the more gradually and gently when the person is poisoned by outside agents and poisoned inwardly. One must understand and accept the crises of toxin ejections set off by the body, without trying to suppress them but helping to get through them intelligently.

When a person makes the effort to acquire good habits and adopt the small, very simple habits, that can be so powerful when they permeate his/her daily routines, he/she will be like an investor who has set aside small sums of money every week and after years of very modest sacrifices is in the position to buy a house or some other valuable, dreamed-of asset.

In this context I should like to mention a great figure[29] in the medical, psychological and literary world, who is also a very human person and of whom, no doubt, all my American (as well as English) readers will have heard, namely, Dr Scott Peck, MD, international best-selling author of The Road Less Traveled (Arrow 1978).[30] In an audio cassette recording, Dr Peck tells how he was asked to prepare a sermon on one of the parables of Jesus, often wrongly interpreted, little understood and even on the face of it shocking to a Christian conscience. This is the parable of the ten wise and ten foolish virgins. They were told in substance: "Be ready, since the long hoped-for Bridegroom may arrive at any moment, and you must not miss this one opportunity!" The ten foolish virgins laughed off the warning. They allowed their lamps to deteriorate and did not think of replenishing the precious oil to keep alive the flame which would be so vital when the time came... As for the ten wise virgins, they got the message and took care to keep their lamps prepared for use and have the oil ready for the special day.

When the day, or rather the night, suddenly came, and they had to join the bridegroom in the darkness, the ten foolish virgins, now completely panic-stricken, implored the ten wise virgins to share with them this light which was to lead them to their beloved. The wise virgins explained to the ten foolish ones that they could not possibly share with them what they had patiently maintained with humility and devotion for so long! " No way!"

Good sense and charity tend to be revolted by this refusal, which seems a priori pretty selfish. However, it is not a question of a refusal, but simply of an impossibility! Let us think, dear reader, a little while about this, and transpose this parable into a context we know well–that of a way of life that respects the Principles of the Laws of Life. Those among us who over the years have tried to follow with determination and sincerity, a way of physical cleanliness and moral rectitude, have built a fortress of health and strength which is our personal possession. Despite all our good will, it is not in our power to transfer this purity, this force and this resistance immediately to anyone. Such an immediate transfer would be a super-human miracle and therefore outside the realm of human capacity.

In the same way, an athlete who trains for months and years cannot transfer his strength and courage to a "dreamer" who participates in sports via the television screen. Or a student who has spent the whole year pre-paring for his exam cannot suddenly transfer his knowledge and know-how to the comrade who has spent that time hanging around bars with the girls–even if he begged him on his knees! The farmer who has spent decades improving his land will have the benefit of fine harvests, while he who has allowed his fields to become choked with weeds will have behaved exactly like the ten foolish virgins and can do no more than harvest the bitter herbs and sour fruits of his apathy and laziness.

To follow the aromatic maintenance program conscientiously and apply the complementary techniques which I have explained, corresponds exactly to the provident attitude of the ten wise virgins. This treasure, reader, nobody will be able to take from you: it is yours for the rest of your life. You cannot impart, attribute or pass it on to someone else, however intense your desire to do so. This seems hard, but it is simply just and fair. The person who has chosen to do nothing to defend his or her health and to strengthen his or her resistance must accept the natural result.

We could also call to mind Walt Disney's cartoon of the "Three Little Pigs." Only the third one had the foresight to build a house solid enough to resist the violent attacks of the hungry wolf. He could momentarily lodge his two unfortunate, or rather brainless, fellows, who had not taken the threat seriously, but after that it was up to each of them to learn to build his own safe shelter. The world at present is dominated by "an industrial and financial wolf," continually hungry for more power and dominion. It is based on the chemical folly that creates the destruction of the exterior environment and the pollution of our "interior milieu." If we do not use our agency and will power to build a protected domain, the probability of developing more "civilization sicknesses" will become ever greater.

The first step then concerns each one of us and our families. We must be aware that the only chance of helping someone else lies in showing them the way to go, encouraging them to move forward and helping them in their difficult moments. This by itself is quite an achievement!

A warning: take each step according to your personal priorities, do not disrupt everything from one day to the next. Experience has taught me that over-enthusiasm and zeal at the beginning fall very quickly and the old habits take over. It is better first to change one or two aspects that seem to have the highest priority and are incompatible with a choice for healthy living (I am thinking especially of the use of tobacco), than to try to take it all on at once, finish nothing and abandon everything. For a reform in depth, it is advisable to feel guided and supported by a professional therapist, who will act like a prop for a freshly transplanted young tree, still fragile in its new home. In our medical practice my wife and I ask that if possible all the members of the patient's family come together for collective apprenticeship on taking control of their health. If only one member of the family undertakes a serious and regular treatment, misunderstandings can set in with the risk of imbalances and frustrations. Since it is often the mother who takes this first step towards a change of life, others in the family tend to talk about a "new sect" as soon as there is a departure from the "well-traveled road." If the husband agrees to accompany his wife and children, he will listen to reason and good sense and be better able to accept a few changes and new habits. As to grandparents, you will have to show authority imbued with respectful but firm diplomacy.

Some advice drawn from my own experience: at the beginning, act without talking too much about it to other people. Once you have acquired practice and know-how, share your experience first with those who ask and are sincerely seeking real solutions. It is quite useless to force anybody on these issues.

If the fruit is ripe, pluck it at the right moment; if the fruit is green, allow it to mature by itself; above all, do not let it rot! You must know that all the aromatic exercises which you believe and which you introduce progressively into your life will lead to a transformation both in you and in those about you. Now that you have read to the end you are different than you were at the beginning. As a writer and teacher, this change and evolution in you are my most valuable reward.

I should like to give my final message for this first book in the form of a scene, which I can see clearly in my mind:

I have before me a very respectable representative in the high quality aromacology and aromatherapy line. He has an impressive range of "absolutely perfect" products and his essential oils are surely "the best in the world." But his ego was all puffed up and his skin particularly thick. His praiseworthy requirements had turned to rigidity and his heart had hardened. As a result of comparative judgements, criticisms, attacks, condemnations, exclusion, "excommunication" even, the small spark of Life had wavered and gone out in the cold. **Even the most biological and purest essential oils can never replace the warmth of light from the small flame that shines in the depths of the heart**.

I turn away from this unhappy vision; I turn around and this time find before me an English style aromatherapist. Is she English, Scottish, Welsh or Irish? Does she come from Canada or the United States? Perhaps she is Australian, a New Zealander or South African? What does it matter? After all, it is not essential. The essential, said St Exupéry, is only visible to the eyes of the heart. My heart feels she wants to talk to me and senses that her message deserves to be known to every man and woman. So I let her talk:

"Dr. Pénoël, I perfectly understand the need to work with the best products available. The fight against mediocrity and in favor of the best quality must be carried on and I am happy to have discovered a whole new world of aromatic practice that I suspected existed and have been seeking for a long time. The story of Abby touched me more deeply than I can say and I know essential oils are the strongest pillar for the medicine of the coming century. I've got with me about thirty essential oils I use for diluted aromatic massages, "ESA" style. I'm not sure these oils correspond exactly to the most stringent qualitative requirements. I haven't been able to get all the necessary technical, botanical and biochemical information on them. But there are three things I am sure of:

1. The sincerity of my intention to relieve suffering,

2. The intensity of my will to do good,

***3. The purity of my desire to give of myself in the act
of aromatic massage,*** *for which I have been trained.*

And in all honesty, Dr. Pénoël, I can tell you I am convinced that these intentions and motivations, this will and desire, count at least as much and often even more, in the help I give my patients, than the intrinsic value of the product employed. I shall in the future use the qualitative criteria I have discovered through reading your book, but I would like you to understand, with all my strength, this ultimate Truth:

> ***In my approach, strength of heart transcends and transmutes the aromatic substance in a spray of light and gentleness which envelopes my patient and finishes by touching the inmost depths of his being. This transfusion of Life and Love and the sharing of the best of myself with the Other are the essence itself of every authentic cure. All these people tormented in body and soul who come to see me, nobody has ever truly held out a hand to them, always in a hurry and more and more reduced to technical performance.***

This intimate relationship which is established between us, this effort which I give and this abandonment of a part of me during aromatic care sessions in the English fashion, "à l'anglaise" as you call it, are the most valuable elements in my work. In this approach the aromatic extracts surely play a subtle and even determining role, but only in so far as all my strength of mind is applied without reserve or calculation in the fulfillment of my work, which is almost a work of alchemy, from the spiritual angle. The essential oil then acts as a catalyst which permits a reaction to take place and develop much more rapidly.

There you are. That's what I wanted to tell you, quite simply, and on the strength of my daily experience, I know and feel we understand each other and basically we talk the same language. Thank you for allowing me to speak at the end of this book; and I fervently look forward to its sequel. We are committed to the same road to the future."

This message is the quintessence of all I have received and perceived on the part of my aromatherapy friends in the English-speaking world. I wanted very specially to share it with you, as an ultimate homage to the memory of all those who have given their lives to passing on the light of their intellectual knowledge, enriched and energized by the warm strength of their loving heart.

If I may leave you with just one more thought, it is these few lines that came to me in English as I meditated beside my "sacred" Juniper tree, facing the mountain of Roche-Colombe:

"Leave the old way

To live the new way,

Learn to forgive,

Accept to receive,

Feel the joy to give,

And, above all,

Live unconditional Love."

Footnotes

28. It sometimes happens that the use of a specific essential oil or well-designed oil blend sets off a process of accelerated "cure" incomprehensible from a conventional medical point of view. An energetic and information-based approach to the human body–physiological and psychological–makes it possible to interpret these real cases which many aromatherapists have come across in their career. I should like to say here that it is important first of all to establish one's aromatherapy practice on a solid foundation of respect for the Laws of Life. In the majority of cases, and Abby is but one example among a hundred thousand others, long hours of hard work and discipline are required in order to obtain authentic results.

29. Among the great figures, in the sense of strong personalities who have transmitted a message capable of transforming millions of lives, I should mention Dr. Wayne Dyer, author of several best sellers. I made his acquaintance through audio cassettes when we were in Melbourne. In my book about our Australian adventure, "The Story Behind the Story," I shall return in detail to this determining "encounter" from a psychological point of view. The revolutionary message he brought to clinical psychology in some ways is similar to the message I transmit through Integral Aromatic Medicine.

30. Dr Scott Peck is also the author of *"People of the Lie"* (1983), *"What Return Can I Make"* (1985), *"The Different Drum"* (1986) and *"A World Waiting To Be Born"* (1993).

RECOMMENDED FURTHER READING

*M*y intention here is to list a few selected books to help the reader in developing a better understanding of aromatherapy, nutrition and personal development. Most books on these subjects are found in health food stores and in the natural health sections of most bookshops.

About essential oils and aromatherapy:

"Essential Oil Safety" by Robert Tisserand and Tony Balacs. (Churchill Livingstone, 1995)

"Aromatherapy for Health Professionals" by Shirley and Len Price (Churchill Livingstone, 1995)

"Clinical Aromatherapy in Nursing" by Jane Buckle (Arnold, 1997)

"Aromatherapy: An A-Z" by Patricia Davis (C. W. Daniel Company, 1988)

"Aromatherapy for Healing the Spirit" by Gabriel Mojay (Gaia Books, 1996)

"Aromatherapy Workbook" by Marcel Lavabre (Healing Arts Press, 1990)

"The Fragrant Pharmacy" by Valerie Ann Worwood (MacMillan, 1990)

"Aromatherapy for Scentual Awareness" by Judith White and Karen Day (Nacsons and Sons, NSW, Australia, 1992)

"Aromatherapy," by Vivian Lunny, MD (Smithmark Publishers, New York, 1997)

About nutrition and natural medicine:

"Fit for Life" by Harvey and Marilyn Diamond (Warner Books, 1985)

"Living Health" by Harvey and Marilyn Diamond (Bantam Press, 1988)

"Diet for a New America" by John Robbins (Stillpoint Publishing, 1987)

"The Missing Link in the Medical Curriculum" by Dr. Jay M. Hoffman, PhD (Professional Press Publishing Co., 1981)

"New Dimensions in Health" *From Soil to Psyche* by David A. Phillips (Woodbridge Press and Angus & Robertson, 1977)

"Vibrational Medicine" *New Choices for Healing Ourselves* by Richard Berber, MD (Bear & Company, 1988)

"Love Your Disease, It's keeping You Healthy" by John Harrisson, MD (from Adelaide) (Angus & Robertson, 1984) (A very interesting book dealing with the psychological basis of physical disease.)

"Superbug, Nature's Revenge" *Why antibiotics can breed disease* by Geoffrey Cannon (Virgin Publishing, 1995)

Several excellent books on health and nutrition written by Dr. N. W. Walker and published by Norwalk Press. Available in most health food stores.

About personal development and global thinking:

All the written and recorded works of Dr. Wayne Dyer, particularly "The Sky's The Limit" (Simon & Schuster, 1980)

All the written works of M. Scott Peck, particularly "A World Waiting to Be Born" *The Search for Civility* (Arrow, 1993)

"Unlimited Power" by Anthony Robbins (Fawcett Columbine, 1986)

"Awaken the Giant Within" by Anthony Robbins (Simon & Schuster, 1992)

"The Path of Least Resistance" *Learning to Become the Creative Force in your own Life* by Robert Fritz (Fawcett Columbine, 1984)

"Super Joy" by Paul Pearsall, PhD (Bantam Books, 1988)

"The Global Brain" *Speculations on the evolutionary leap to planetary consciousness* by Peter Russel (J.P. Tarcher, 1983)

"The Turning Point" by Fritjof Capra (Simon & Schuster, 1982)

"The Wholeness Principle" by Stephano Sabetti (Life Energy Media, 1986)

"Parallel Thinking" by Edward du Bono (Penguin Group, 1994)

Complexity, *Life at the Edge of Chaos* (J.M. Dent, London & Macmillan, USA, 1993) A major new theory that unifies all sciences.

PRESENTATION OF THE CD AND ROSE PRINTEMPS METHOD

A Tribute from Dr. Pénoël to His wife

*A*romatic plants, their essences and music have a number of similarities. Rose-Marie, under her pseudonym of Rose Printemps, lives only through and for creation. Whether working in her "culinary laboratory," or counseling those who come for her help, or caring for children animals, and plants, or taking up her pencil or brush to produce book covers or CD jackets, the creative impulse reigns supreme in giving deep meaning to her life.

Above all, in a gift of ultimate creative harmony, Rose-Marie gives herself in song and movement. In the act of singing, every fiber in her being, every chord in her soul, each pearl that falls from her heart and every flame that lights up her spirit all join together in unison to sing of joy, gratitude, respect, harmony, confidence, generosity and love. This Love of Creation, of creatures and their Author, Rose-Marie carries to fulfillment in this first "Rose-Printemps" CD.

Each composition tells its own story. Music and words melt in a melodious synergy which, for those who are receptive, works deeply and subtly as a musical therapy in the highest sense.

Each of the eight major compositions corresponds to a vibratory levels (Chakras) of the human body. This led to the idea of ascribing to each a gemstone and an aromatic composition. The "Rose Printemps Method" is born of this musical, mineral and aromatic alliance, which can further the work of reharmonizing and balancing the world surrounding us. The medicine of the twenty-first century will help us realize that vibratory phenomena contain the keys for understanding sickness and health. Music and aromatic substance, in depth, echo the subtle harmonies that contribute to our well-being and the opening of our personality. It is therefore only right that this complementary step should be included in the global osmobiotic method.

Rose-Marie is available to help therapists or private individuals sensitive to this approach with more information, as a counselor and as a seminar leader.